HON

with

YOUR BODY

HONORING GOD
with
YOUR BODY

What the Bible Teaches
Us about Wellness

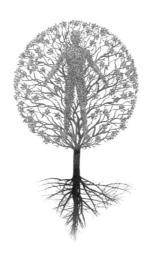

R. PRICE FUTRELL

Published by Happy Self Publishing
www.happyselfpublishing.com

Table of Contents

PSALMS 139:1-16 (PFV)[1]

Father God,
You have thoroughly examined me from top to bottom and You know exactly who I am.

You know when I stand up and when I sit down. You always know what I'm thinking.

You see me as I go about my day and when I come home to rest. There isn't anything that I do that You aren't completely aware of.

You know what I'm going to say even before it comes out of my mouth.

You surround me with Your presence, and we connect.

It is so very difficult to comprehend the magnitude of who You are.

Where could I go that You couldn't find me? A place that Your spirit cannot go?

If I were to travel into the heavens, you would be with me. Into the depths of the earth, you would find me.

I could rise upon the wings of the morning or dwell at the bottom of the sea, and even there Your hand would lead me, and Your right hand would protect me.

I was worried that darkness might hide me from You: Complete darkness where there is no light.

But there is no such thing as darkness to you. To You, darkness and light are the same. You can see equally well in both.

You designed and created my body in my mother's womb.

I praise you and stand in awe when I think of how incredibly meticulous and with such craftsmanship you created me. My entire being knows how incredible your works are.

Nothing was hidden from You as I was being created in my mother's womb.

You saw my unformed body and already knew what my life was going to look like, even down to the very days of life.

I don't know how one could read the above passage and not get an intense and overwhelming sense of God's love for us. Despite knowing everything there is to know about who we are and where we're headed with all our emotional and spiritual warts, He loves us! He knows that we are fragile creatures. He knows how much we struggle to get it right. Perhaps it is because He designed us to be like we are: Dependent upon our Father's love to survive, that He loves us so.

There is difficulty in writing such a book as this. There is difficulty in speaking to what the Bible says about protecting one's health from the front of the congregation on Sunday mornings. You most likely haven't heard it discussed in your Bible study groups either. Living a healthy lifestyle is difficult to discuss when there are people in the pew or seat beside you who haven't yet mastered the art of being disciplined about their health.

One can preach on and have study classes on lying, cheating, stealing, drunkenness, adultery, etc., and we can identify no one as being guilty of these indiscretions simply by their appearance in church or, if you prefer, the assembly. Unfortunately, that's not the case with being fit or unfit. So, we don't talk about it out of a sincere concern that we might offend someone.

Oh, but not the thief or the liar. We don't mind offending them because we don't know who they might be. They are the unknown sinners of whom we speak and whose actions we lash out against. And if the Word says we shouldn't do it, then the church is obligated to inform its members. Except when it comes to health and wellness.

The likelihood that you've heard a Sunday morning sermon on what the Bible says in its entirety on God's instructions, preferences, and admonition regarding our well-being is not very high. And so, we tacitly approve of inappropriate behavior by not speaking the truth in love.

People are dying at a record pace from the self-inflicted wounds of poor life choices. It's neither the acceptable standard of the life we were designed for nor an appropriate reflection of God to the world. We're covering our influence and "light" with the bushel of destructive personal habits, and that must change. It must change for the good of the people and the impact and influence of the church.

How many of you would be offended if the preacher stumbled to the pulpit in an inebriated state? How many would tolerate a church leader who was having simultaneous sexual encounters with people other than their spouse? How many would continue to allow a church member to assist in counting the contributions if they were caught unapologetically stealing the money? But we accept as normal, joke and laugh about, and encourage those who are literally committing a slow and painful suicide that is spoken so very plainly against in the word of God.

But rather than come up with another "fire and brimstone" teaching, we must understand our weaknesses and try to love each other back toward the ideal. We can't do that very well with shame and condemnation. So, not only do we present what the truth is from the pages of inspired text, we offer information, techniques, and solutions for EVERYONE, including those with genetic and medical challenges, to provide hope and reassurance that each of us can live a more abundant life even though life is, at times, unfair.

Foreword

GOD, The Master of Prevention and Healing.

The goal of this book is not one of condemnation, shame, or disgrace. Nor is it an attempt to suggest one must look like the pro body builder or fitness competitor on the cover of the magazine. Nor is it an attempt to create yet another trip hazard on the proverbial slippery slope into the fires of Hell. No, the goal is to provide an understanding of the intentional design of wellness for our lives as outlined and described in the inspired words of scripture.

The Faithful believe GOD cares about our health. How can this be so assertively stated? Well, first of all, GOD has told us HE cares. Heck, nearly fifteen percent of GOD's directions for the Israelites contained within the Law of Moses concerned their health. Secondly, we all have as individuals and corporately in our assemblies lifted up prayers of healing and/or recovery on behalf of friends and family members concerning some aspect of their health. If we didn't believe GOD cares about our health, why would we petition HIM concerning it?

GOD was and is all about prevention, scripture is clear. No different from any parent, GOD has given us guidance and admonition on what to do and what to avoid in order to maintain our good health. Scripture clearly indicates that poor health was most often the result of failure to adhere to these instructions or as a punishment for other moral failures. Good health and wellness maintenance were the original design.

"And Jesus increased in wisdom and in stature and in favor with God and man." (Luke 2:52, ESV) Mentally, Physically, Socially and Spiritually, we are to emulate our Savior and strive toward improvement. If we drop the ball in one area, it has a deleterious effect on the other dimensions of our being as they are all connected. How many times have I seen a person get way off track in their physical well-being which leads to poor self-esteem, people avoidance, and a stressed relationship with their Lord? More than one might imagine!

> *"All scripture is given by inspiration of God, and is profitable for doctrine, for reproof, for correction, for instruction in righteousness: That the man of God may be perfect, thoroughly furnished to all good works."* (2 Timothy 3:16-17)

All scripture is given by inspiration of God. In the Greek language, the word that we translate ALL... means ALL. Given that the New Testament, as a whole, wasn't written at the time of Paul's admonition to Timothy, we know that his reference to "scripture" was what many today would consider the "Old Testament." Some might wish to emphasize that we are no longer condemned by the Law, but one would be foolish to disregard the instructions of how to live a life of good health. The original design hasn't changed. We got an Owner's Manual on how to treat the only machine ever designed to repair itself, and we best pay attention!

Here are a few examples of scripture addressing the wisdom of paying attention.

> *"Let the wise hear and increase in learning, and the one who understands obtain guidance."* (Proverbs 1:5)

The wise don't turn a deaf ear to instruction. They listen to those with understanding and apply it in their own lives, and they continue to build upon their successes. Don't let your ego, or excuses, get in the way of self-improvement; that is, you becoming the best version of you possible.

One of my favorite sayings is this: "No fool is ignorant." A "fool" isn't lacking instruction. They are lacking the good sense to follow that instruction. If you know better, do better, otherwise you've made yourself into a fool.

> *"The hand of the diligent will rule, while the slothful will be put to forced labor."* (Proverbs 12:24)

Lazy folks don't make it happen. Don't settle for mediocrity. Don't become complacent. If you find yourself wishing you felt better, had more energy, slept better, weren't carrying around all that extra weight, then you have to be diligent with your effort to change. Complaining, making excuses, blaming others for where you're at hasn't helped and won't ever help you get to where you need to be. Take back your authority over your life by accepting responsibility and do the do!

You can't get to the top of **your** ladder without climbing the rungs.

> *"Leave the presence of a fool, for there you do not meet words of knowledge."* (Proverbs 14:7)

This proverb could easily have said leave the presence of the undisciplined, or the one who, in any area of their life, lacks self-control. Avoid people that encourage ill-advised behavior. Stick with people who challenge you and encourage you to grow in every aspect of your life; physically, mentally, and spiritually.

"Whoever loves pleasure will be a poor man; he who loves wine and oil will not be rich." (Proverbs 21:1)

The reason that video games are so popular is that they give us a sense of accomplishment with little effort. Be wary of things that reward you for little work. Don't give in to short-term temptations, but invest in the long-term.

"Like a dog that returns to his vomit is a fool who repeats his folly." (Proverbs 26:11)

Mistakes are inevitable; we all are going to make them. Every once in a while you are going to "get off the rails," finding yourself in the ditch. But when you do, learn why that happened and resolve to never do it again. The fool is not the one who makes a mistake, but the one who continually makes the same mistake without learning from it. Living a lifestyle daily, which damages our physical, mental, or spiritual health, is like the dog returning to its vomit.

These are just a few scriptures, inspired words of GOD, from Proverbs. Each and every word addresses the way to live from a physical, mental, and spiritual perspective

You are about to embark on a journey through the word of God as it relates to His intent for our well-being. These passages with examples and admonitions are not often discussed and yet they should be so that the "man (and woman) of God may be fully equipped for every good work and a shining light for the world to see."

In Good Health,
Stephen Ashcraft
President, Cor-Restor
https://www.cor-restor.com
stephena@cor-restor.com

CHAPTER ONE

The Admonition

In much of our study of biblical writings, cultural context is of paramount importance to our understanding. Knowing how society influenced a person's daily life gives us insight into the admonitions, commands, and prohibitions often ascribed to that time. Understanding the context gives us much-needed insight into how we are to apply the principle or specifics of certain passages in our lives today. Paul told Timothy that, "All Scripture is breathed out by God and profitable for teaching, for reproof, for correction, and for training in righteousness" (2 Tm 3:16, ESV[ii]). Knowing how to do that properly is important to us if we are to live the abundant life that God wants us to live. Sometimes the context is clear, sometimes not so much, so we need to be cautious and studious in our approach.

As an example, most of us understand that we are not under obligation to necessarily "greet one another with a holy kiss," [1] as was the admonition to the Romans or to have all the men raise their hands when they pray.[2] We also understand

---

[1] Rom 6:16
[2] 1 Tm 2:8

and accept that Paul's instruction to Timothy to speak out against women who braided their hair or wore pearls was a statement against what was considered inappropriate and immodest dress **at that time in that culture**![3] If you look at Ezekiel 16, most of the things Paul tells Timothy to put a stop to, God symbolically adorns Jerusalem with as a special honor! He even adds a nose ring! Obviously, it was a different time and culture! And, while I'm not a fan of tattoos personally, one would be hard-pressed to use the time and culture of the 1400s BC in Leviticus 19:28 to make a case for their prohibition. Clearly, it is the **principle** of the admonition that speaks from those ancient times.

Yes, regardless of cultural norms, we can use the instruction principle in the above passages to understand that in any culture, one should dress modestly. Men and women should treat each other honorably. Christians should set themselves apart and avoid imitating immoral and decadent images in present-day society. One need not get off into the weeds of the specifics to understand the overarching principles that would apply to our lives today if we accept the premise that godly principles will endure beyond any cultural norm.

An overarching summary of the topic discussed shows how the Bible relays timeless principles. An example of this type might be in how Jesus summed up the whole Mosaic Law and the writings of the prophets:

> *"Teacher, which is the great commandment in the Law?"* [37] *And he said to him, "You shall love the LORD your God with all your heart and with all your soul and with all your mind.* [38] *This is the great and first commandment.* [39] *And a second is like it: You*

---

[3] 1 Tm 2:9

shall love your neighbor as yourself. [40] *On these two commandments.*" (Mat 22:36-40, ESV)[iii]

Amazing! Just two key principles were the foundation upon which God based all the countless laws and regulations! This summation of loving God and loving our neighbor and ourselves is as helpful in answering our questions about what would be the best thing to do or to avoid as it ever was. We don't have to know all the answers if we understand the key principles upon which God bases the answers.

In 1 Corinthians 6, Paul addresses the Corinthian church and leadership regarding various judgment errors in the church. He addresses how people should avoid using the judicial system to mitigate disputes among members and avoid immoral behavior and sexual promiscuity, which was pervasive in their culture. In fact, the whole book is a unique letter of back-and-forth dialogue between Paul and the church leadership, addressing a whole host of questions they had and concerns that Paul had because of his people reporting back to him what they observed while there. And besides these great truths, it is in this chapter that the Holy Spirit gives us an eternal principle, an admonition that will guide us in any culture, in any time, or in any setting without having to address a specific issue: Honor God with your body (1 Cor 6:20$_b$).

Now, I've heard some people attempt to disqualify this overarching admonition by relegating its application to, and only to, sexual immorality. I don't believe that's true at all. Yes, sexual immortality is definitely the topic at hand, but the admonition to "honor God with your body" is the foundation upon which we base the command to avoid sexual immorality. It's true to life as we know it.

3

When your parents told you that you couldn't buy the bubble gum because they didn't want you to waste your money, they didn't mean you could buy the candy bar. Not wasting your money was the principle that you were to understand. When they told you to get down out of that tree because they didn't want you to fall and hurt yourself, they weren't giving you permission to climb up on the side of the house. When they told you not to play in the street because they didn't want you to get run over by a car, they weren't giving you permission to play in the street when no cars were present. I know—I learned that one the hard way. Back in my day, you didn't give some lousy excuse to justify your disobedience without severe consequences. My folks didn't know about "time out." So how does this apply today?

To my knowledge, cigarettes didn't exist back in the first century. Does the absence of a command to avoid smoking make it OK? Knowing what we now know about smoking and the deleterious effect on one's health, one could hardly say that smoking is honoring God with your body. Does the absence of a command to avoid abusing pharmaceutical drugs make it OK? What about other recreational drugs common in our culture? What about eating or drinking excessively to the point of ill-health and disease? I guess one could debate the true meaning of gluttony and its correlation to obesity, but my guess is that you'd be trying to point out the difference between climbing way up in a tree versus climbing on the roof of the house. When we get off into the weeds of debate, we miss the spirit of the admonition!

But how do we know that God cares about how we treat ourselves? What are the admonitions, if any, that identify overarching principles that affect us today? Well, let's look at scripture and see if it tells us anything that we may not have noticed that could give us a clear sign.

CHAPTER TWO

In the Beginning: Created by Design

And God said, *"Behold, I have given you every plant yielding seed that is on the face of all the earth, and every tree with seed in its fruit. You shall have them for food"* (Gen 1:29). If it were a plant or a fruit that could be grown from seed, it was designed as nourishment for humans. Humans were designed to receive appropriate nourishment from certain plants and fruits. This is to say: our nourishment was, and is, by design.

It is possible to live a healthy lifestyle if you eat a 100% vegetarian diet. Many do. It is from plants (what we commonly refer to as vegetables) and fruits that we can get our vitamins, minerals, trace minerals, and the energy sources of protein, carbohydrates, and fat that fuel our human existence. The nutritional value of these original plants, grown in original dirt, in original purified air, must have been amazing. Can you imagine how good that first homegrown tomato was?! But my how things have changed.

We know that plants and veggies get their nutritional value from the soil. Good soil = good plant. Poor soil = poor plant. Unfortunately, the nutritional value of plants that most people consume today has been substantially depleted due to profit-motivated farming practices (Davis). Commercial growers have been interested in growing larger and better-looking fruit and veggies to appeal to the consumer in the most cost-effective means possible in order to sustain the growing operation. You can't be a farmer for very long if you can't make money doing it! Pesticides, herbicides, and fungicides became popular, and their widespread application introduced poisonous chemicals into the soil, which were taken up into the plant and ultimately into our bodies. What we discovered is that the chemicals that killed the weeds also significantly harmed the soil. The microorganisms that God designed into the soil to help break down the plant's minerals were killed by these chemicals. As a result, it broke the chain of soil to plant, plant to man nutrient transfer.

It's reported that most of the soil in the United States is contaminated by these chemicals (Pesticide Use in U.S. Agriculture). It has also been demonstrated that we have had a significant decrease in the nutritional content of fruits and vegetables. One can understand why the "organic" market has grown so much in the last couple of decades. But organic, according to the organization that certifies items as being such, doesn't mean nutritious or completely free of these chemicals (Laufer). Wow! We've come a long way in many areas of human development, but how we produce our food for consumption has been focused almost entirely on quantity rather than quality, with very little regard for nutritional value.

At some point in early human development, we began eating meat. Some suggest that it was not until after the flood due to their understanding of Genesis 9:3: *"Every moving thing that lives shall be food for you. And as I gave you the green plants, I give you everything."* People who believe that Adam and his family only ate fruits and vegetables could be quite right, but I've always thought it strange that Adam and his family would raise flocks of sheep if they didn't eat them. There are lots of other animals to have as pets than a smelly ol' goat!

Everybody knows the story of Cain and Able and how Cain's offering wasn't acceptable, but Abel's was. Genesis 4:4 says, *"… and Abel also brought of the firstborn of his flock and of their fat portions. And the LORD had regard for Abel and his offering."* Apparently, Able even knew how to clean and process the sheep to present the good portions as an acceptable offering to God. It seems that he cooked it for God too. So perhaps they raised them, slaughtered them, and knew how to cook them—and yet didn't eat them—but that doesn't sound plausible to me. Later, God gives Moses instructions in His Laws to avoid certain animals and fish that were not very healthy to eat. Lizards, frogs, and stuff like that were off-limits, as were catfish and shrimp. I know, right?

Regardless, it was early on that man began consuming certain animals' meat, which added another dimension to the nutrient content, particularly regarding amino acids, which form what we commonly refer to as a protein molecule.

Unfortunately, just as in the commercial production of vegetables and fruits, we see some of the same influences in raising animals for food. To sustain and increase profits, producers used antibiotics to ward off disease and hormones and other stimulants to rapidly increase growth rates (Chemical Use in Animal Production: Issues and Alternatives). As with plants, the synthetic and chemical treatments given to the animals transferred into the bodies of those that ate the meat. This includes adults **and** children.

So, we see that man was designed to eat certain plants and animals and that these plants and animals were designed to be consumed by humans to provide life-sustaining nourishment. We've also seen how commercial production has messed it up by contamination of soil and the heavy use of chemicals in food production to increase profits. Obviously, it's in our best interest to consume the cleanest and most uncontaminated foods possible.

CHAPTER THREE

Note to Noah

Interestingly, not every instruction by God to man is detailed in some special way: We just find out about it. Such is the case regarding "clean" versus "unclean" animals.

> *"Take with you seven pairs of all clean animals, the male and his mate, and a pair of the animals that are not clean, the male and his mate . . ."* (Gen 7:2).

> *"Then Noah built an altar to the LORD and took some of every clean animal and some of every clean bird and offered burnt offerings on the altar"* (Gen 8:20).

This is the first time in scripture that clean and unclean animals come up. Unless we assume that God gave an instruction which was impossible for Noah to understand, we must assume that there was, at some point, a directive from God to man that outlines what a clean animal was and was not. We don't see Noah being confused and asking God to define clean and unclean, so apparently, he knew.

If we jump ahead to the Mosaic Law, specifically Leviticus 11, God gives detailed instructions regarding the eating of clean and unclean animals. However, this may have been the official recording of rules and regulations that were already delivered to early man that we don't have a record of. Perhaps it was amended in some way beyond the previous instructions. Some have estimated that there are roughly 2,500 years between Adam and Moses, and at least by Noah's time, people were aware of what was clean and unclean. Maybe not so much by the time they were leaving Egypt. We don't know what the original instructions included; we only know by some reasonable assumptions that there were instructions before the Law was created. But we do know **some** of the instructions.

> *"Every moving thing that lives shall be food for you. And as I gave you the green plants, I give you everything. But you shall not eat flesh with its life, that is, its blood"* (Gen 9:3-4).

Here we must be careful in realizing what God said and what at first glance we might **think** He said. Some say that God permitted Noah to eat all animals, except they needed to be prepared properly (no blood). But is He saying that? I don't think so because of the qualifying statement "as I gave you the green plants…"

And God said, *"Behold, I have given you every plant yielding seed that is on the face of all the earth, and every tree with seed in its fruit. You shall have them for food"* (Gen 1:29). Did God say it was OK to eat all plants? No. Just the ones that produced seed. The rest was for some other purpose besides human consumption. So, when God says, "just as I gave you the plants," it is a qualifier for the type of animals that could be eaten. God gave them an outline of what should be considered eatable and what shouldn't (clean/unclean) and then perhaps He elaborated on it further in the Law.

All we know for absolute certain is some things are not good to eat! Let me repeat that. Since the beginning ... by design ... mankind was created in such a way as to benefit physically from the consumption of certain plants and animals, but **only** those certain plants and animals. And physical harm would result from eating anything that wasn't supposed to be eaten. The same is true today.

CHAPTER FOUR

Manna, Quail, and Nutrient Timing

"I have heard the grumbling of the people of Israel. Say to them, 'At twilight you shall eat meat, and in the morning, you shall be filled with bread. Then you shall know that I am the LORD your God'" (Ex 16:12).

Everybody pretty much knows the story of how the Israelites were grumbling about the lack of food, and God, rich in mercy and probably running out of patience, provided additional selections on the menu. Manna in the morning for breakfast and quail for supper. I guess you were on your own for lunch, which is the very first sign in history that there is, in fact, no such things as a free lunch.

Read how manna is described in Exodus: *Now the house of Israel called its name manna. It was like coriander seed, white, and the taste of it was like wafers made with honey* (Ex 16:31). Since nobody knows exactly what manna was, and there isn't any remaining to examine, we can only guess what it was made of and what sort of nutrient content it had. But, according to the 31st verse, it tasted like wafers (bread) made with honey. It was, according to the description, sweet. It sounds like a divine breakfast cereal to me. The sweet taste indicates that it may have been a source of carbohydrates, like sugar, which is an energy source for the body when eaten in moderate amounts. Wandering around in the desert probably required considerable energy resources, so God not only responds to their grumbling with food, but He provides a nutritious and energy-packed meal to begin the day. Being God undoubtedly makes Him the best nutritionist ever! But that wasn't all.

In the evening quail came up and covered the camp (Ex 16:13$_a$). Quail for dinner! Now that's awesome. Anybody that has ever eaten quail knows that it is one delicious meat. It is also high in protein and low in calories and carbohydrates. A whole quail (anybody could eat one) is around 135 calories and has approximately 22 grams of protein and **zero** carbs. It is ideal for an evening meal. It has a low amount of energy (carbohydrates), and it's rich in nutrients, especially protein, which provides the ingredients necessary for weary muscle recovery.

But of course, the Israelites had no idea of what a calorie was. They didn't measure protein. They knew nothing of vitamins, minerals, and the like. They didn't know about nutrient timing or about how what you eat and when you eat it affects the body. However, it's clear from what science has taught us about these things is that, most assuredly, God knew. Yep, God is the Great Nutritionist. He knows how to properly feed His people when it's His turn to fix the meal.

So, we know that God is a patient and loving God. From this event we can also learn something that nobody ever talks about: The timing of using certain foods makes a big difference! And, quit skipping breakfast! It's the most important meal of the day, but you need to do it right (Cho). Consume higher carbohydrates in the morning to meet the day's anticipated energy demands and then much lower in carbs with lean protein for recovery overnight. Many people today will skip breakfast on the way out the door and then overeat at supper and add dessert on top. That's exactly the opposite of how God, who knows best about the creation, designed it. And maybe, just maybe, you don't need to eat 2,000 calories at lunch either. Perhaps a snack would do.

CHAPTER FIVE

The Law of Moses

It has been determined that there are some 613 different "laws" outlined in the Mosaic Law. It has been estimated that approximately 14% of these laws have to do with the preservation and protection of life. That's quite a focus on health! Perhaps we should pay attention.

Dietary restrictions in the Law were very direct. Here is a list:

- Do not eat any unclean animal. (Dt 14:7-8)
- Do not eat any unclean fish or seafood. (Lv 11:10-12)
- Do not eat any unclean fowl. (Lv 11:13)
- Do not eat any unclean flying insect. (Lv 11:20-23)
- Do not eat any insects that creep on the ground. (Lv 11:41)
- Do not eat any reptiles. (Lv 11:44)
- Do not eat worms found in fruit or produce. (Lv 11:42)
- Do not eat any swarming insects. (Lv 11:43; Dt 14:19)
- Do not eat any animal found already dead. (Dt 14:21)
- Do not eat a torn or mauled animal. (Ex 22:31)

- Do not eat any meat with the blood still in it; neither eat any meat not fully cooked. Only when meat is cooked until it is white inside with no tinge of red or pink whatsoever ensures that all blood had been removed. (Dt 12:23)
- Do not touch the carcass of an unclean animal. (Lv 11:8)
- Do not eat blood. (Lv 7:26-27)
- Do not eat the meat of a bull that has been stoned to death for goring someone. (Ex 21:28)
- Do not partake of drink offerings to the gods (false gods). (Dt 32:38)
- Drunkenness of any sort is prohibited. (Dt 21:20)

Now I don't know about you, but I'm not into eating worms or lizards, but at some point in human understanding and development, we needed instruction on what parts of God's creation could be used as food. As far as it can be determined, these instructions regarding health issues were the first formal ones to be articulated and transcribed by God. We can see from just a cursory reading that the preservation of life and the avoidance of disease, ill-health, and death were important to Him. So much so that He gave very direct and specific instructions that included severe penalties for the failure to observe them. God was serious about people paying attention to their health.

Proper hygiene needed to be maintained. It was important to avoid even touching something that could be diseased. It was important to avoid eating plants and animals that weren't designed to be consumed by humans. It was important to respect the health of someone else. It was important to isolate and quarantine infectious individuals. There is no way to read these instructions in the Law and not see the significance God placed on good health—unless you weren't looking for it.

Where I'm from in the southern part of the USA, folks would have a problem with some of these instructions. Catfish would be outlawed. You know how much catfish is consumed in the South! Shrimp, oysters, and even buzzards are on the do not eat list as well. Why? They are all bottom feeders, devouring diseased and rotted flesh. These are filtration and debris organisms, the trash dumps of nature. In other words, they clean up the environmental garbage by consuming it, and if you eat them, you eat the garbage. The worse the environmental filth, the worse it is to consume. In fact, there are warnings and advisories issued by the Department of Natural Resources literature that warns against eating more than a certain amount of fish from the rivers and streams in all 50 states!

Ancient Israel didn't know about the dangers of swine brucellosis, pseudorabies, or parasitic disease. God did. The dangers that existed in 3,500 BC still exist today. Most, if not all, of the warnings God gave Israel are as applicable today as they ever were! We would do well to pay attention to the dietary instructions and warnings in the Mosaic Law, not because they judge us but because we are instructed and protected by them!

CHAPTER SIX

Two Fat Men

If your name is in the Bible, you are immortalized. Your name is likely to be mentioned from time to time for as long as people study the word. If your name is Abraham, Isaac, Jacob, Moses, Joshua, David, Isaiah, or Paul, you probably feel pretty good about how you got mentioned. If your name is Judas . . . not so much. Some are remembered for their great faith and deeds. Others are remembered for less than complimentary reasons. I don't know about you, but I would rather be remembered for calling fire down from heaven as did Elijah, or even for turning my life around like the prodigal son, than I would for being some reprobate or heathen. And, if I was not a total reprobate or heathen, being less than what I should have been would be a bad enough way to be remembered. But, to add the unfavorable description of me as fat to my already inappropriate conduct and character would be downright embarrassing! Thus, the remembrance of Eglon and Eli.

EGLON, KING OF MOAB (JUDGES 3:12-25)

As usual, the Israelites found themselves in trouble with God because they couldn't seem to pay attention and do what was right. So, God empowered Eglon, along with the Ammonites and Amalekites, who then captured the Israelites at Jericho (City of Palms) and forced them into captivity and servitude for 18 years. Then, as was usual for God, He saw His kids suffering and had pity on them and raised up a guy named Ehud, from the tribe of Benjamin, to take on ol' King Eglon. For some reason, the biblical account takes the time to mention that Ehud was a lefty. One can only wonder why the writer identified Ehud as being left-handed, since there is no seemingly apparent reason for mentioning it. Perhaps it was to point out how accurate the writer was with the detail of the story.

To make a short story even shorter, after some special ops and conniving on Ehud's part, he thrust a homemade, two-edged sword into the belly of Eglon. The writer takes the time to give us a lot of detail and indicates that Eglon was so large that his belly fat overlapped the blade jammed into his stomach. The rest of the details are kind of gross, but suffice it to say that this was the end of ol' Eglon.

It's interesting to notice the facts chosen to be immortalized in this story. Not only do we know that Eglon was the king of an anti-Israel heathen nation, but it was apparently necessary to point out that he was extremely obese! And not just really, really fat, but that he was so fat that all that flab completely covered up the hilt of the sword that Ehud stuck into his abdomen. I'm pretty sure that everybody would agree that this wasn't a compliment.

ELI, HIGH PRIEST AND JUDGE (1 SAMUEL 1-4)

Before we talk about Eli, I think it's important to remember that first and foremost, this was a man of God and due respect should be given to him. He was a Judge and Prophet. That's a lot of responsibility and a clear sign that God thought a good bit of Eli. I think it's a big mistake to ignore a man's life work and focus on nitpicking his shortcomings. Who among us could withstand such scrutiny?

It's also a mistake to overdo a critique of a story and try to pull a teaching moment out of a passage that was never intended to be one. The fact that Jesus found Zacchaeus up in a sycamore tree versus an oak tree has nothing to do with the point of the narrative, so we need to be careful. At the same time, it is a mistake to miss all that the story teaches, even if it is not the primary point of the narrative. The primary message of Eli seems to be the concern God has for not taking seriously the responsibilities that He gives us and allowing ourselves, and those for which we may have oversight, to become complacent or negligent. But there is another message which we shouldn't miss, which may relate to this idea of complacency and neglect.

The first mention of Eli is in Chapter 1, verse 9. He's sitting down. The last mention of Eli is in Chapter 4, verse 19, and he's once again sitting down. I guess we can assume that Eli liked to sit. One wonders why?

Chapter 2 describes Eli's sons as generally worthless. They hoarded portions of the sacrificial meat and even threatened those coming to offer their sacrifices to take even more. They ignored their priestly duties in the most callous of ways, including inappropriate contact with the women that hung out around the church building. The entire community was upset by what they were doing and how they conducted themselves. And yet Eli did nothing. Well, mostly nothing.

He at least asked them why they were being so stupid, but he never stood up and exercised his authority to stop his sons' nonsense. He never called on God, as far as we know, to help him stand up to the ignoble conduct. Perhaps he should have done less sitting on his behind and gotten up to be the man that had propelled him into being Judge and Priest, but alas, he just sat down. And God was **not** happy about it.

But being merciful as He is, God sent some unnamed person to tell Eli that calamity was about to happen in a big way because of his sons' conduct and because of his acquiescence toward and participation in it. The story could have ended with such a great ending if Eli had gotten off his duff and took care of business, but apparently, he never did. So, what was the main issue that this unnamed person tells Eli?

*"Why then do you scorn my sacrifices and my offerings that I commanded for my dwelling, and honor your sons above me by **fattening** yourselves on the choicest parts of every offering of my people Israel?"* (1 Sm 2:29) There it is: Disrespect and Gluttony. It was bad enough that Eli was allowing his sons to disgrace the office of Priest and doing nothing to stop it, but he was also taking part by gorging himself on the sacrificial meat that they inappropriately obtained. Eli had more of a priority on his appetite than he did on God, and God wasn't happy about it. Which, by the way, is fairly obvious since God sent some unknown person to speak to Eli instead of having a personal conversation with him. The guy had been a Prophet and Judge for 40 years, and now God shuts down

one-on-one communication. Nope, not happy at all. So, what was in store for Eli?

For one thing, the sons were toast. That is to say, for those unfamiliar with "toast" as a colloquial expression, they were going to die—that same day. And as far as the legacy of being a Priest, Eli and his family would no longer be honored in such a way. That was a **big** deal. His family would forever be remembered in disgrace. Sad. But then God had to throw in one more little parting shot.

> *"And everyone who is left in your house shall come to implore him for a piece of silver or a loaf of bread and shall say, 'Please put me in one of the priests' places, that I may eat a morsel of bread'"* (1 Sm 2:36).

In other words, no more pigging out on quality food for you or your family tree. You're done getting fat off Me. In fact, generations after you will know what it's like to be hungry. Ouch!

Sure enough, the Philistines engage Israel in battle and kill 30,000 men and capture the Ark of the Covenant. Eli's sons are killed in battle, and Israel is totally defeated. When word of the battle's result reaches Eli, he falls off his chair and breaks his neck from the fall because he was old and heavy.

Listen to the last comment . . . the epitaph of Eli . . . the etching on his tombstone for all time; for an old Judge and Prophet who enabled and took part in the dishonoring of the priesthood . . .

Here lies Eli—"for he was old and FAT."

CHAPTER SEVEN

Fat, Fatter, Fattest

[15]But Jeshurun grew fat, and kicked; you grew fat, fatter, and greatly fat; then he forsook God who made him and scoffed at the Rock of his salvation. [16]They stirred him to jealousy with strange gods; with abominations they provoked him to anger. [17]They sacrificed to demons that were no gods, to gods they had never known, to new gods that had come recently, whom your fathers had never dreaded. [18]You were unmindful of the Rock that bore you, and you forgot the God who gave you birth (Dt 32:15-18, PFV).

We all have a beginning and an end. After being called a friend of God and leading the Israelite people through some of the most trying times, the chairman of the board says it's time for Moses to turn over the corner office to a new CEO.

After commissioning Joshua, God does something unusual, which is so like God, who makes the unusual usual: He dictates to Moses a song to teach to the people.[1] The Song of Moses. Pretty neat.

---

[1] Dt 31:19

In this song, God laments that the people of Israel will swerve off the straight and narrow path and do all sorts of stuff that they shouldn't and provoke Him to anger. In this song that they are to memorize and teach to their children, God uses a <u>metaphor</u> to describe their progression of disobedience. He says that they have grown fat (*Shaman*), gotten even fatter (*Abah*), and have covered themselves in fat and became obese (*Kasah*). That's how it happens.

One doesn't go from a loyal follower to totally disobedient overnight! One doesn't get obese overnight! It is a progression of inappropriate behavior patterns that develop into a lifestyle. But, don't you think it's telling that God uses the process of getting fat to describe the process of becoming disobedient? It's not as though the Israelites had to be taught that growing fatter and fatter until one was morbidly obese was something to avoid. It's just that God used it to describe how getting off track a little and ignoring the consequences can lead to an overindulgence, and they understood what He was talking about.

They could have noticed that their faithfulness and passion for God had dwindled and tried to rekindle the flame, but they didn't. They became lazy and content in their abundance, and as Chapter 31:20 indicates, they turned away from being focused on The Provider and were, instead, only focused on His provisions, to the point they were content, well-fed and fat. Which is to say that they abused their provisions.

There's nothing wrong at all with enjoying the provisions that God so richly provides, but at some point, you need to metaphorically, and in a very literal sense, put the fork down!

CHAPTER EIGHT

Holy Fat Shaming

. . . ²⁶running stubbornly against him with a thickly bossed shield; ²⁷because he has covered his face with his fat and gathered fat upon his waist (Jb 15:26-27).

Nothing like having friends! For those familiar with the book of Job, we know that God is trying to fix something in Job and uses Satan to assist unknowingly in the effort. After considerable crisis and physical pain has been inflicted, Job's friends come to the rescue. But instead of comforting him, they blame Job for behavior that has brought calamity upon him and his household.

In this particular passage, Eliphaz the Temanite is giving Job the dickens by suggesting that Job is bearing the consequence of his sinful behavior. Eliphaz's description of Job as needing a big shield to cover his fat body is a put-down on Job as having so much sin to cover that he needs a big shield to deflect attack.

Now whether that has any truth to it at all isn't the point. It's that growing fat is used as an example of defiance and stubbornness toward proper behavior. Being obese is used by Eliphaz as a metaphor of accumulated sin. It is widely accepted that the characters of Job are of ancient descent and one of the earlier times recorded in biblical history. From the beginning, being fat was looked down upon as a dereliction of duty to care for oneself properly.

> [23] *But this people have a stubborn and rebellious heart; they have turned aside and gone away . . .* [28] *they have grown fat and sleek. They know no bounds in deeds of evil; they judge not with justice the cause of the fatherless, to make it prosper, and they do not defend the rights of the needy* (Jer 5:23, 28).

God is once again angry at the misdeeds and willful disobedience of His people and verbally lashes out against them. Part of the description of their disobedience and neglect is, besides the focus on ill-gotten prosperity, that they have overindulged and become fat in the face of others' apparent need in the community.

God wants you to have an overflow of good things, but there is a limit. Overindulgence and gluttonous behavior is never looked upon favorably.

> [6] *Therefore pride is their necklace; violence covers them as a garment.* [7] *Their eyes swell out through fatness; their hearts overflow with follies* (Ps 73:6-7).

Asaph, the author of this Psalm, is lamenting his own envy and jealousy toward the success of others. Not just "others" but those he describes like this: For I was envious of the arrogant when I saw the prosperity of the wicked.[1]

They are "living the dream," and he's had a tough time with comparing his lifestyle with theirs, which is one of

---

[1] Ps 73:3

great prosperity and overindulgence! They've enjoyed great prosperity of which he is jealous, but then he throws out an insult: they've gotten so fat that their eyes are about to bug out of their face! Wow! Even in the ancient world, being extremely obese was negative. He probably shouldn't have mouthed off, but God let it go through to print.

CHAPTER NINE

The Real Health Lesson of Daniel

³*Then the king commanded Ashpenaz, his chief eunuch, to bring some of the people of Israel, both of the royal family and of the nobility,* ⁴*youths without blemish, of good appearance and skillful in all wisdom, endowed with knowledge, understanding learning, and competent to stand in the king's palace, and to teach them the literature and language of the Chaldeans.* ⁵ *The king assigned them a daily portion of the food that the king ate, and of the wine that he drank. They were to be educated for three years, and at the end of that time they were to stand before the king.* ⁶ *Among these were Daniel, Hananiah, Mishael, and Azariah of the tribe of Judah.* ⁷*And the chief of the eunuchs gave them names: Daniel he called Belteshazzar, Hananiah he called Shadrach, Mishael he called Meshach, and Azariah he called Abednego.*

⁸*But Daniel resolved that he would not defile himself with the king's food, or with the wine that he drank. Therefore, he asked the chief of the eunuchs to allow him not to defile himself.* ⁹*And God gave Daniel favor*

and compassion in the sight of the chief of the eunuchs, [10]and the chief of the eunuchs said to Daniel, "I fear my lord the king, who assigned your food and your drink; for why should he see that you were in worse condition than the youths who are of your own age? So you would endanger my head with the king."

[11]Then Daniel said to the steward whom the chief of the eunuchs had assigned over Daniel, Hananiah, Mishael, and Azariah, [12]"Test your servants for ten days; let us be given vegetables to eat and water to drink. [13]Then let our appearance and the appearance of the youths who eat the king's food be observed by you, and deal with your servants according to what you see." [14]So he listened to them in this matter, and tested them for ten days. [15]At the end of ten days it was seen that they were better in appearance and fatter in flesh than all the youths who ate the king's food. [16]So the steward took away their food and the wine they were to drink and gave them vegetables (Dn 1:3-16).

Now, **this** is the real example of Daniel: Not some once-in-a-while or beginning-of-the-year fast to feel good about doing briefly what Daniel and his buddies regularly did! Yeah, everybody has probably heard about the "Daniel Fast." It happens every January. Millions of people go on some partial fast and then go right back to whatever they were doing previously. That's **not** what the example of Daniel is about.

Daniel and his buddies, Hananiah, Mishael, and Azariah, were the young, smart, good-looking, healthy, and articulate members of the captive Jews. Shadrach, Meshach, and Abednego were their slave names and were the names we, unfortunately, taught the kids in VBS. Hananiah, Mishael, and Azariah are what their mommas named them. They were the best of the best and were being groomed to integrate into Babylonian society by their captives. The head man in charge had three years to get them ready to stand before the king as a finished product. In a sense, it was a Babylonian Boot Camp.

It was probably a much better existence than what the rest of the captives were facing. They were being treated well and even had their meals prepped just like the king wanted! They were living relatively "high on the hog," as we say back where I grew up. But there was one problem: Daniel and his buddies couldn't stand the food.

Remember, Jewish dietary rules and restrictions were very specific. And here, Daniel and the gang were forced to eat fried chicken with mashed potatoes and gravy, sweet tea to drink, and banana pudding for dessert! Well, that's not exactly what it was, but it wasn't what they were comfortable eating, according to their upbringing. They didn't like the wine either. Not that Jews had any problem drinking wine, but maybe they were serving it for breakfast, or a little too often. Whatever the reason, they knew it wasn't good for them, and they decided that they weren't going to eat any more of it. So, Daniel went to the man in charge.

Scripture says that Daniel was given favor with the guy. That's important when you complain about what kind of food you're being served when you're a prisoner. But Daniel also showed excellent judgment in how he handled the situation. He let the boss know that they didn't like the food and wanted something else. Of course, the boss wasn't exactly thrilled and worried that they would look all puny before the king, and he might suffer the consequences, so

Daniel offered up a challenge.

Daniel said, "Let us do what we know is good for us for ten days, and you compare us with the rest of you Babylonian boys, and let's see how we compare!" Since God had intervened and given Daniel favor with the guy, he agreed. Daniel, his buddies, and perhaps all the rest of the young Jewish men asked for and were given veggies to eat and water to drink. That's not a fast. That's a lifestyle change. So, how did it turn out?

Ten days later, they compared the groups, and Daniel and the rest were visibly superior. Their appearance improved, and their bodies were "more firm" (Bariy'). Various translations often use the word "fat" as a translation of the Hebrew here, but another definition of the word which can be used, and is used, is **firm**. I believe that's more accurate. You don't get fat eating veggies and drinking water: You lose fat. And when fat is removed your muscles start to show and you look noticeably healthier. In fact, the boss was so impressed with the comparison he made the change permanent for the Jewish boys. One must wonder if some Babylonian guys didn't get in on it as well. Why look less than your best if you could look all fit and buff?

I think it's most important to emphasize that this was **not** a fast. They were going to be in prep mode for three years, and this was the new menu. This was not some twenty-one-day fast, but rather a total change in lifestyle. That's the lesson of the first chapter of Daniel. But that's not to discount fasting as a health benefit.

Fasting is good. Medical science has informed us about how beneficial fasting can be if nutritionally supported for a very brief period. Fasting helps the body kick into overdrive relative to flushing out toxins and impurities and increasing human growth hormone (HGH), but it is not a substitute for proper eating habits. If we learn anything from Daniel's example, let it be that we, anybody, can change our physical appearance and our underlying health in a brief period if we decide to eat healthily.

It's also interesting to notice that God only intervened in giving Daniel favor with the Babylonian boss when he requested to change the menu. Scripture never infers that the physical results of Daniel and the rest were miracles by God. It was a natural result of eating what the Creator designed us to eat. What's the takeaway? You can change your physical appearance, just like Daniel, if you change what you eat, just like Daniel.

CHAPTER TEN

Bless This Food to the Nourishment of Our Bodies

When you spread out your hands, I will hide my eyes from you; **even though you make many prayers, I will not listen**; *your hands are full of blood. 16 Wash yourselves; make yourselves clean; remove the evil of your deeds from before my eyes; cease to do evil* (Is 1:15-16).

You ask and do not receive, *because you ask wrongly, to spend it on your passions* (Jas 4:3).

If I had cherished iniquity in my heart, **the LORD would not have listened** (Ps 66:18).

. . . but your iniquities have made a separation between you and your God, and your sins have hidden his face from you so that he **does not hear** (Is 59:2).

We know that God does not listen to sinners, *but if anyone is a worshiper of God and does his will, God listens to him* (Jn 9:31).

Whoever closes his ear to the cry of the poor **will himself call out and not be answered** (Prv 21:13).

If one turns away his ear from hearing the law, **even his prayer is an abomination** (Prv 28:9).

They made their hearts diamond-hard lest they should hear the law and the words that the LORD of hosts had sent by his Spirit through the former prophets. Therefore, great anger came from the LORD of hosts. "As I called, and they would not hear, **so they called, and I would not hear***," says the LORD of hosts* (Zec 7:12-13).

Therefore, thus says the LORD, Behold, I am bringing disaster upon them that they cannot escape. **Though they cry to me, I will not listen to them** (Jer 11:11).

There they cry out, but he does not answer, because of the pride of evil men. **Surely God does not hear an empty cry***, nor does the Almighty regard it* (Jb 35:12-13).

*They cried for help, but there was none to save; they cried to the LORD***, but he did not answer them** (Ps 18:41).

Then they will cry to the LORD, **but he will not answer them***; he will hide his face from them at that time, because they have made their deeds evil* (Mi 3:4).

What do you see in these verses? I see an unwillingness by God to answer the prayer of those that have no genuine interest in doing what is right.

God has given us instructions on how to take care of ourselves. So, what are the odds that He's going to answer your request to "bless this food to the nourishment of our bodies, and our bodies to Thy service" if what you are consuming is in blatant disregard of His instructions? Slim to none?

Some would argue that Paul tells Timothy that prayer makes all food OK. Let's see . . .

For everything created by God is good, and nothing is to be rejected if it is received with thanksgiving, for it is made holy by the word of God and prayer (1 Tm 4:4-5).

First of all, Paul is **not** saying that the dietary laws are obsolete and that eating lizards is OK. And secondly, a cheesecake isn't made by God. Look on the label of the food item: If you see more man-made than God-made, it's not real food. Some of the junk food that people eat . . . wow. Asking God to bless that is absurd. Do you honestly think eating rat poison won't kill you?

Occasionally I get pushback from people who try to claim that they can't afford to eat according to the instructions. Really? God has told you what to do, and you are unable to do it? Have you asked for His assistance? Why can't you afford it? Is it because you've ignored a bunch of other instructions that got you in a financial hole? A reasonable person might concede that there would be an occasion when there weren't any options and that the prayer would be a sincere request. But we all know better. Just about anybody can afford to eat better, but they first must make it a priority.

Consequences are rarely the result of coincidence. You might want to underline that.

The bottom line is that God will not bless manufactured fake food with little to no nutritional benefit any more than He's going to make sure you don't get hurt when you decide to jump off the top of a twelve-story building. In fact, it seems a little insulting to thank God for something He doesn't want you to do.

Now, before you think of every exception—just don't go there. Surely God would bail you out in an emergency, but testing God regularly because I'm hardheaded isn't on my bucket list and shouldn't be on yours.

CHAPTER ELEVEN

Just Because You Can, Doesn't Mean You Should

"All things are lawful," but not all things are helpful. "All things are lawful," but not all things build up (1 Cor 10:23).

The translators' quotations let us know that "all things are lawful" was a statement or position statement from the Corinthian church. They had been taught and firmly believed that God didn't condemn Christiana for what they did in walking out their daily lives. Yet, Paul offers a practical, timeless, and universally applicable response to the theological complexities of grace.

Paul rebuts their position by saying that not all things are helpful and not all things build up. Wow! Is that a great response or what! Yes, you can avoid condemnation for doing something technically not a "sin," but does it make the situation better? Does it encourage and uplift the people around you? Is it good for you?

Is it a sin to have banana pudding? No. Is it a good thing to serve around people who are obese and struggling with weight issues? No.

Is drinking a sin? No. Is it a good thing to serve around recovering alcoholics? No.

Is smoking an occasional cigar going to send you to hell? Probably not, but is it a good thing for the preacher to do on the church's front steps on Sunday morning? Not according to Sister Wilbanks.

Can you eat what you want and not feel condemned? I suppose. But is it helpful? What does it do to your health? Does it set a good example? Are you honoring God with your body?

See? There's more to it than just being technically accurate. There's the impact and influence of what you do.

CHAPTER TWELVE

Knowing Better

Come on, you know better than that!

Have you heard that before? Usually it involves an incredulous response to an action or expression of intent that is seemingly void of logical thought. Not uncommon around teenagers! Most of the time, it's relatively easy to know whether you should or you shouldn't, and if you shouldn't . . . don't!

> *So whoever knows the right thing to do and fails to do it, for him it is sin* (Jas 4:17).

The use of the Greek word, hamartia, which is translated to "sin," seems to mean the negative consequences or result of doing something you know better than to do versus some eternal condemnation to hell. It just means that you're messing up. You're squandering the opportunity to do the right thing, and you know better. You should aim to hit the bullseye, but you missed the whole dartboard. You get the point.

One flaw of religious, well-meaning people is making everything that isn't technically correct a matter of condemnation to hell. It is a **SIN** in bold capital letters, and those doing it should be shamed and shunned. The Old Testament Hebrew uses six different nouns and three verbs to describe sin. The New Testament Greek uses five nouns, five adjectives, and three verbs. When one considers all the various words used for "sin," we realize that not everything is a major big deal. Some things are just not recommended if you're looking for a good outcome.

This verse is another great example of an admonition that crosses over every cultural barrier for all time. If you know better than to do it . . . don't do it. If you know better, do better. Pretty simple. If you go ahead and do what you know isn't right, you're messing up and might experience an outcome that you would have preferred to avoid. No, you might not be condemned to eternal punishment, but what you're about to experience might feel like it!

Nowadays, you'd have to have your head stuck in the sand not to have a basic understanding of what you can and can't do to live in good health. It's not that you don't know. If your bad health is self-inflicted, it's that you don't care. You look in the mirror and see what everybody else sees—that you've got 50 pounds of extra and unnecessary fat hanging on your frame, and so far, you've done nothing but make excuses. Come on! You know better than that! Figure out what's going on and do something different.

To be fair, we didn't know what manufacturers of food-like products were doing to our food to influence our purchasing habits. We didn't know they added that much sugar. We didn't know how addictive sugar was. We didn't know that they were using preservatives that **caused** fat gain. We didn't know they were using other chemicals that cause cancer and other issues. And if you don't know, you can't be held responsible, right? Well, maybe it's not your fault per se, but most of us can tell if we've gained 50 pounds and might have prediabetes with high blood pressure. Come on!

How many times have companies been told to stop selling products because of the false claims associated with them? You thought you were getting some health benefit from an included ingredient that was practically nonexistent. How long are you going to believe everything you hear on TV or read on the Internet? Come on man!

Did your physician tell you to push away from the table and get some exercise? Worst advice ever. You're eating food with little nutritional value, and the medical advice is to eat less? On top of that, you're to ask your body to perform outside the norm? Horrible advice. But then again, keeping you in a state somewhere between healthy and dead is where the money is made in medicine.

If what you don't know will kill you, then it's in your best interest to know. Actually, it's your obligation and responsibility to know. You are responsible for yourself! And if you're a parent, you have the responsibility to guide those youngins as well! And once you know, the admonition is for you to do the right thing. I don't know how it could be made much simpler than that.

CHAPTER THIRTEEN

Love Your Neighbor "As Yourself"

"And a second is like it: You shall love your neighbor as yourself" (Mt 22:39).

One must conclude that when written, it was assumed that each person would have a high regard for oneself! It can only be assumed that the average person wasn't trying to harm themselves intentionally by their daily habits—my, how things have changed.

Obesity levels have risen to about 40% of the adult population. Childhood obesity is just over 30%! How can that be? Somewhere around 60% of all sickness and disease is directly attributed to our dietary habits. That's nuts. We are committing suicide. Just because death isn't immediate makes it no less self-inflicted. I know some will object to that statement. But is suicide defined by how soon the result is realized? If you are knowingly doing things that will cause you to die, does it matter how long it takes?

Would I want to be your neighbor if I was forced to experience the impact and effect of your lifestyle? No way! Would I want you to love on me like you're loving on yourself? Hardly.

CHAPTER FOURTEEN

Drunkard and Glutton

*. . . and they shall say to the elders of his city, 'This our son is stubborn and rebellious; he will not obey our voice; he is a **glutton and a drunkard**'* (Dt 21:20).

*. . . for the **drunkard and the glutton** will come to poverty, and slumber will clothe them with rags* (Prv 23:21).

*The Son of Man came eating and drinking, and they say, 'Look at him! A **glutton and a drunkard**, a friend of tax collectors and sinners!' Yet wisdom is justified by her deeds"* (Mt 11:19).

*The Son of Man has come eating and drinking, and you say, 'Look at him! A **glutton and a drunkard,** a friend of tax collectors and sinners!'* (Lk 7:34).

God doesn't mind if you drink alcohol so long as:

- You don't think it's something you shouldn't do and do it anyway.
- It causes somebody else to make poor decisions (stumble).
- You do it to excess.

God doesn't mind if you drink alcohol so long as (a) you don't think it's something you personally shouldn't do and do it anyway, (b) it causes somebody else to make poor decisions (stumble); or (c) you do it to excess. That's about the same restrictions placed on eating.

Paul said that eating meat offered to idols isn't a good thing to do theologically, but if you're with friends and you're not sure where the meat came from, you might just not ask. Better for your conscience to not know, and then you don't mess up your dinner plans and embarrass your host. Not likely to happen today, but you get the overall message. Other than restrictions on eating stuff like lizards and buzzards, the only real admonition associated with eating is don't be an overeater!

Now let's stop right here for just a second to dispel an uncommon excuse that I've heard offered up, which is that gluttony is eating to the point of puking and then eating some more. Or, gluttony is how one eats (gulping it down). Hogwash. Gluttony is an overindulgence of food. Being drunk is an overindulgence in alcohol. Neither eating food nor drinking alcohol is wrong, but doing so in excess is a problem.

What I find interesting is that each time gluttony is specifically named, it is directly associated with drunkenness. Now how many preachers and upstanding women of the church would be offended if the majority of people that walked into the assembly on Sunday morning were drunk? How many in the assembly are **obviously** gluttons? Are we saying that shouldn't matter?

I can feel the blood pressure rising. But let me ask you a question: Is it OK to avoid teaching the truth of scripture because many people are guilty of not acting right by it? Is it OK to not speak the truth because most of the people who put money in the plate are doing what you need to teach against? Why don't we teach about it? I have never heard a sermon on Sunday morning about being a glutton. Never. And I get it.

You can't look around the assembly and quickly notice the liar, the guy cheating on his wife, the thief, or the woman who drinks too much. These sins aren't outwardly noticeable. But when we change to talking about the overindulgence of food. Well, some folks—more like 2/3 of the audience, will be offended, embarrassed, and ashamed. And it's a great way to be encouraged to find another preaching job. I get it. It doesn't make it right, but I get it. But surely there is a time and place to speak the truth in love about this subject. And perhaps it will give us some pause to consider how we speak and condemn other "sins" that we don't do (supposedly) and the impact on those that are listening who are struggling.

I know people who will stand up at every available opportunity to rail against homosexuality—in the assembly and online. And none of these people have ever stood up or gotten online to condemn obesity, and many of them are, in fact, obese. Why is that?

Let me be perfectly honest: If you're a fat preacher, I have a hard time listening to anything you have to say. Why should I listen to somebody about being a disciplined person if you are not? What you are saying is probably accurate, but because you have a visibly obvious problem with gluttony, I don't want to hear you stand up and tell us what we ought to do, much less condemn the actions of somebody else. It's hypocritical. It's wrong.

Unfortunately, the church in its acquiescence has become the greatest encouragement of sinful eating habits. Several studies showed that in North America, the more often a person attends worship services per week is an indicator of whether they are likely to be obese (Gillum) (Dodor). Have you seen what we serve at the potluck dinners? I notice that there isn't any liquor, beer, or even wine served, but the high carb, less-than-nutritious food-like substances, along with Ms. Magnolia's banana pudding on a whole other side table of desserts, is common. Why? Because we don't take obesity seriously. In fact, we encourage and promote it. So, yeah, I don't listen to fat preachers.

Gluttony, the overindulgence of food, is wrong. Period. There are serious consequences to ignoring the instruction manual on this issue, the least of which is "going to hell." It's probably not a "hell" issue unless you consider living in a state of disease a "living hell." It's a "living the life as you were intended to live, free of sickness and disease" issue. It's a "now" issue. It's a "witness" issue. It's a "testimony" issue. It's a "look at me; I live for Jesus" issue. That's the truth you should have been taught from the front of the room on Sunday morning.

CHAPTER FIFTEEN

But Jesus Said I Could Eat Anything I Want

Uh . . . no, He didn't. But rather than throwing that out there as an opinion, let me see if I can make the point. Here is the passage that some use to declare that it's OK to eat anything you want.

> [18]*And he said to them, "Then are you also without understanding? Do you not see that whatever goes into a person from outside cannot defile him,* [19]*since it enters not his heart but his stomach, and is expelled?"* *(Thus, he declared all foods clean.)* (Mk 7: 18-19)

Here is the parallel passage recorded in Matthew: *Do you not see that whatever goes into the mouth passes into the stomach and is expelled? But what comes out of the mouth proceeds from the heart, and this defiles a person."*[1] Notice that there is not a declaration of all foods being clean as there is in the passage from Mark.

---

[1] Mt 15:17-18

There are few reasons that I believe "Thus, he declared all foods clean" was a scribal addition without divine inspiration:

1. It's not in the earliest of manuscripts as presented.

Codex Sinaiticus or "Sinai Bible" is one of the four great uncial codices, ancient, handwritten copies of the Greek Bible. The codex is a celebrated historical treasure. The codex is an Alexandrian text-type manuscript written in uncial letters on parchment in the 4th century (Wikipedia contributors). The Codex Sinaiticus translation says "making all meats clean" instead of the parenthetical entry, "Thus, he declared all foods clean." Obviously, the digestive process and elimination of the food doesn't make the elimination clean. That's nonsense. But what Jesus meant is that the normal process of the body is designed so that any impurities that enter the body through the consumption of food (the outside) that might be present from not washing one's hands are eventually removed from the body. The nourishment remains, but the impurities are discarded, leaving the body protected from the impurities. The meat is "cleaned" by the digestive process, and the impurities are separated out and discarded.

2. The scribal addition indicates that the person didn't understand the message. Food wasn't the subject under consideration.

The issue at hand is the objection raised by the Pharisees that Jesus wasn't making sure that His disciples followed the Jewish traditions of only eating after properly washing their hands. Jesus then compares the physical impurities that enter the body and are removed to that of spiritual impurities which emanate from inside the body and corrupt the person. He further explains:

> *²¹For from within, out of the heart of man, come evil*
> *thoughts, sexual immorality, theft, murder, adultery,*
> *²²coveting, wickedness, deceit, sensuality, envy, slander,*
> *pride, foolishness. ²³All these evil things come from*
> *within, and they defile a person (Mk 7: 21-23).*

3. The same account in Matthew doesn't mention any declaration that the Law was being altered to include "unclean" meat as now clean.

That would have been a **big deal**! The Pharisees were blowing a gasket just over the lack of proper handwashing, which was a tradition and not part of the Torah. Imagine their outrage had they understood that Jesus was declaring the dietary laws of the Mosaic Law to be void! Scripture wouldn't have been able to avoid their outrage. It's evident from the text that they did not understand him to be saying that "unclean" foods, as outlined explicitly in the Law, were now "clean."

4. The actions of the Jerusalem council would have conflicted with this declaration.

As you might recall, what is commonly known as the Jerusalem Council (Attending Apostles, Elders, and other members of the congregation there in Jerusalem) met to work out an issue with Jews and Gentiles in this new era of all men being accepted by God. Specifically, they wanted to work out how to interact with one another at mealtime. Eating with someone was to accept them as a friend and brother—a fellow heir. Some of the Gentile converts were raised where they would buy and eat the meat offered to idols, and some preparation customs violated clearly stated Mosaic Law. So, they sat down and came up with this solution, which seemed good to all involved: *that you abstain from what has been sacrificed to idols, and from blood, and from what has been strangled, and from sexual immorality. If you keep yourselves from these, you will do well. Farewell* (Acts 15:29).

As seen in Deuteronomy, not eating anything raw that still has the blood in it is specifically forbidden in the Law: *Only you shall not eat the blood; you shall pour it out on the earth like water* (Dt 12:16). *Only be sure that you do not eat the blood, for the blood is the life, and you shall not eat the life with the flesh* (Dt 12:23). The prohibition against eating an animal that had been "strangled" was another tradition, as it is not specifically mentioned in the Law. It was probably one of the clarifying instructions the Jews used to correctly interpret the specific Law's intent. Nonetheless, it was included in the agreement of the association to appease the conscience of the Jews. But, if **all** food was now "clean," then the Jerusalem Council didn't understand Jesus' declaration as they would not have put any restriction on any type of food.

5. Peter was adamant that he not consume "unclean" food years after this declaration.

There is quite a bit of uncertainty about how many years had transpired between the death of Jesus and Peter's experience with Cornelius and his household. But it's fair to say that it was some length of time. As you recall from the story of Cornelius' conversion, Peter was given a vision to prepare him for the encounter. Obviously, this was Peter's first foray into a Gentile conversion.

In the dream, Luke records that in Peter's vision, a huge sheet descended from heaven with all sorts of animals in it. Then he hears a voice telling him to rise and eat. Here we are, some years down the road from Jesus' preaching, with one of the closest disciples to Him, who gets a divine command to rise and eat, and he says this: *But Peter said, "By no means, LORD; for I have never eaten anything that is common or unclean"* (Acts 10:14). **Never** has he eaten anything unclean, he says. **Never**! Why would one of the closest disciples to Jesus be adamant about defending his behavior of not eating unclean meat if Jesus had approved it?

Next, in Acts 11, scripture records Peter being called in on the carpet in Jerusalem to explain what's going on with him and the Gentiles and he's asked to explain himself. Which he does here:

> *4But Peter began and explained it to them in order: 5 "I was in the city of Joppa praying, and in a trance I saw a vision, something like a great sheet descending, being let down from heaven by its four corners, and it came down to me. 6Looking at it closely, I observed animals and beasts of prey and reptiles and birds of the air. 7And I heard a voice saying to me, 'Rise, Peter; kill and eat.' 8But I said, 'By no means, LORD; for nothing common or unclean has ever entered my mouth'"* (Acts 11:4-8).

His defense of being a righteous Jew and follower of Jesus was that he had never eaten—not at any time in his entire life—anything unclean. Not a single person at this high-level meeting of Apostles and Elders corrected him by pointing out that Jesus said that it was OK to eat unclean meat.

6. Jesus did not intend to abolish the rules.

> *17 "Do not think that I have come to abolish the Law or the Prophets; I have not come to abolish them but to fulfill them. 18For truly, I say to you, until heaven and earth pass away, not an iota, not a dot, will pass from the Law until all is accomplished. 19Therefore, whoever*

relaxes one of the least of these commandments and teaches others to do the same will be called least in the kingdom of heaven, but whoever does them and teaches them will be called great in the kingdom of heaven" (Mt 5:17-19).

It's evident from a review of the text that neither the Pharisees nor any of the Apostles or other leadership, nor Peter, who was in the inner circle of Jesus, understood that Jesus had approved eating unclean meat. The scribal error is obvious from a total misunderstanding of the text. Jesus didn't change the Mosaic Law's dietary restrictions. If He did, He didn't do it very effectively because **nobody** understood that He did it. Nobody!

CHAPTER SIXTEEN

Lust and Discipline

For everything in the world—the lust of the flesh, the lust of the eyes, and the pride of life—comes not from the Father but from the world (1 Jn 2:16).

[16]But I say, walk by the Spirit, and you will not gratify the desires of the flesh. [17]For the desires of the flesh are against the Spirit, and the desires of the Spirit are against the flesh, for these are opposed to each other, to keep you from doing the things you want to do. [18]But if you are led by the Spirit, you are not under the law. [19]Now the works of the flesh are evident: sexual immorality, impurity, sensuality, [20]idolatry, sorcery, enmity, strife, jealousy, fits of anger, rivalries, dissensions, divisions, [21]envy, drunkenness, orgies, and things like these. I warn you, as I warned you before, that those who do such things will not inherit the kingdom of God (Gal 5:16-21).

Epithymia—a Greek word translated by the King James Version as "lust" and translated by the English Standard Version as "desires." A good present-day translation might be "craving."

There's an old saying, "whatever you can't control, controls you." If you can't put it down, turn away, say no, or otherwise resist the temptation to do whatever it is, you are not in control of your life. You are controlled by a craving, a lust, or a desire, and that's not healthy. Nor is it something that our Creator desires.

As you see in the 1 John passage above, the cravings of the flesh are not from the Father. The Galatians passage shows us how the pure can be perverted. Yes, we were created to want to have sex, eat food, drink water, be happy and sad, be afraid, need companionship, etc., but we were not created to be undisciplined and out of control. Somebody once said that the devil could take anything good and turn it into something bad.

Most people believe that the responsible consumption of alcohol is completely permissible. But we are taught to avoid consuming too much. Procreation is essential to our survival, but we are taught to avoid fornication and sexual perversions. We can't exist without food, but it's clear from the biblical narrative that overconsumption is something to avoid.

Usually when we can't control something, either physically or mentally, the medical professionals refer to it as an addiction. But in all fairness, we didn't know early on that alcohol was addictive. We just thought it was a lack of discipline, and many folks suffered because they didn't get the appropriate treatment. Nobody knew, except the companies that produced them, that cigarettes contained nicotine that was highly addictive. Like, who knew sugar was so addictive? And these addictions are **powerful**!

Unfortunately, most of us know a family member, friend, or

close associate who has been treated for addiction. It often takes extensive intervention and close supervision of medical personnel to have a successful outcome. Abuse caused some of the addictions, and others resulted from individual body chemistry that just happened to be extremely susceptible. But we have an answer.

The first response is kind of obvious, which is to avoid the problem in the first place. Don't drink, don't smoke, and don't do drugs is something we've all heard from early on in life. Avoidance is undoubtedly the best solution to a potential problem. But we don't listen. In fact, as it regards food, we listen to some of the worst advice ever given.

How many of us were told to "clean our plates?" We all heard the stories of children who were starving in some far-off land and that it was wrong to take all this food for granted. Furthermore, there would be no dessert unless you finished. "You can't have any pudding if you don't eat your meat." So, we were taught at a young age to gorge ourselves so we might have a little ice cream. As adults, we can't resist an "all-you-can-eat buffet." Having an endless supply of food to recreate that gorged feeling from our youth has become a favorite marketing ploy. We condition ourselves to eat more than we need and, just like alcohol or drugs, the more we do, the more it takes to get the same effect. How close to the "cravings of the flesh" can this be?

Parents need to **stop** teaching this bad habit. Teach portion control. Teach about dense nutrition. And by dense nutrition, I mean eating things with extensive amounts of vitamins, minerals, and trace minerals per calorie. Stop eating low nutrient, high-calorie food-like substances, and for heaven's sake, quit giving it to your kids as a reward!

In families where one parent is obese, there is a 50% chance that the children will be obese in their lifetime. Where both parents are obese, the odds increase to 80% (Obesity).

The Bible provides another effective solution in the text of 1 Corinthians 9:27: But I discipline my body and keep it under control, lest after preaching to others I myself should be disqualified.

As previously discussed, you can't often discipline yourself out of an addiction without professional help, but you can discipline yourself, post-recovery, to avoid going back. It's also important to note that Paul saw that an undisciplined person who couldn't control themselves was disqualified from preaching to somebody else about being disciplined and under control. If you're fat, you have no business teaching anybody about anything unless you're moving in the opposite direction. Think about it: Would you want a drunk preacher teaching you about avoiding sexual immorality? Hardly.

> *Not many of you should become teachers, my brothers, for you know that we who teach will be judged with greater strictness* (Jas 3:1).

CHAPTER SEVENTEEN

Self-Discipline and Leadership

²⁵Every athlete exercises self-control in all things. They do it to receive a perishable wreath, but we an imperishable. ²⁶So, I do not run aimlessly; I do not box as one beating the air. ²⁷But I discipline my body and keep it under control, lest after preaching to others I myself should be disqualified (1 Cor 9:25-27).

⁷For an overseer, as God's steward, must be above reproach. He must not be arrogant or quick-tempered or a drunkard or violent or greedy for gain, ⁸but hospitable, a lover of good, self-controlled, upright, holy, and disciplined (Ti 1:7-8).

Older men are to be sober-minded, dignified, self-controlled, sound in faith, in love, and in steadfastness (Ti 2:2).

No temptation has overtaken you that is not common to man. God is faithful, and he will not let you be tempted beyond your ability, but with the temptation he will also provide the way of escape, that you may be able to endure it (1 Cor 10:13).

. . . for God gave us a spirit not of fear but of power and love and self-control (2 Tm 1:7).

Whoever is slow to anger is better than the mighty, and he who rules his spirit than he who takes a city (Prv 16:32).

A man without self-control is like a city broken into and left without walls (Prv 25:28).

⁵For this very reason, make every effort to supplement your faith with virtue, and virtue with knowledge, ⁶and knowledge with self-control, and self-control with steadfastness, and steadfastness with godliness, ⁷and godliness with brotherly affection, and brotherly affection with love. ⁸For if these qualities are yours and are increasing, they keep you from being ineffective or unfruitful in the knowledge of our LORD Jesus Christ (2 Pt 1:5-8).

²²But the fruit of the Spirit is love, joy, peace, patience, kindness, goodness, faithfulness, ²³gentleness, self-control; against such things there is no law (Gal 5:22-23).

¹¹Beloved, I urge you as sojourners and exiles to abstain from the passions of the flesh, which wage war against your soul. ¹²Keep your conduct among the Gentiles honorable (excellent), so that when they speak against you as evildoers, they may see your good deeds and glorify God on the day of visitation (1 Pt 2:11-12).

re some passages or other examples left out of this list? Perhaps, but—heavens to Betsy—is this not enough to demonstrate the point? There is absolutely no shortage of material for a wonderful sermon on self-control, isn't there? So, why does it only apply to things which we don't do?

As a practical application of these admonitions in the real world, allow me to tell a quick true story. One of the Brooklyn Dodgers' owners decided that he would do something unthinkable (at the time) and hire a black baseball player on his team. The year was 1947, and African American citizens were not especially welcome just about anywhere. To integrate major league baseball was a tremendous risk to the league, the team, and his reputation, but Branch Rickey was a visionary.

He saw tremendous talent in Jackie Robinson that he believed would improve the chances of his team winning the pennant and the World Series. He also saw a highly competitive man who would likely (and did, in fact) experience tremendous racism and bigotry. In anticipation of that and knowing that Jackie's response to the challenges would matter more than his play on the field, Mr. Rickey wrote a statement that Jackie had to agree to before signing him on to the team. In my opinion, the most significant part of his admonition to Mr. Robinson was this statement: "Only he who has conquered himself is able to conquer his enemies." If Jackie had not been diligent in following this admonition, he likely would have succumbed to the threats and shameful bigotry and reacted poorly to them. This would have ruined not only his professional career but also potentially the careers of those that would follow in his footsteps. The limit of control is within the boundaries of our skin. But God has given us the power to control ourselves. Unfortunately, we don't talk about it much.

I have **never** heard a sermon from the pulpit on a Sunday

morning about obesity in my lifetime. Never. Every other sin known to humankind is addressed, but not that one. And yet, 75% or more of the audience is struggling with this issue. Maybe even the guy in the pulpit!

Paul said that if he didn't discipline his body, he felt like it would diminish his message. He referred to it as being "disqualified." If you have a self-control problem, what business do you have telling somebody else how they should be disciplined and self-controlled? How can you speak about resisting temptation? I don't see how you have any credibility at all. And let's not stop with preachers.

If you're in a leadership role in the church, you must act like it. Titus makes it clear that you must demonstrate self-control. Are you eligible to be considered for a leadership role? Have you disqualified yourself from leadership? Tough question. But lest any of us get on our high horse, scripture admonishes us all!

Did you see the list above? Older men should lead in this area by example! We should "make every effort" to exercise self-control to keep us from "being ineffective or unfruitful." Do you exemplify the Spirit's fruits? Have your emotional and physical walls been so broken down that you are left in an obvious desolated state? No, it's not at all a "leadership" issue: It's an **everybody** issue.

God knows that it's nearly impossible for us to resist certain things. He created us. He's the Manufacturer. He knows how we operate, and He knows where we tend to break down. So, He has promised us that when faced with the temptation to do something that we know we ought not to do— whether it's a lust of the flesh, lust of the eye, or something associated with the pride of life—He will provide a "way of escape." A Door #3; An alternative to select. The only requirement on our part is that we choose.

Life is a series of choices. You didn't "end up" this way; you chose to be this way. What does scripture say? *For as he thinketh in his heart, so is he (Ps 23:7).* You decided, on purpose, to be who you are. You were what you once believed; you are what you presently believe; you will become what you choose to believe. Those are the facts. Your road might have been more difficult than somebody else's, but you made **your choices**. God didn't say He'd only provide for those traveling on smooth surfaces. He promised that **you** would have a **choice** to do what was right. There are some areas of your life where your choice isn't obvious, but then there are those choices that are obvious to everybody. Your choice is your choice. Choose wisely.

CHAPTER EIGHTEEN

Raise 'Em Up Right

Train up a child in the way he should go; even when he is old, he will not depart from it (Prv 22:6).

When you read this verse, what is the first thing that comes to mind? Instruct a child properly, and they will, eventually, do the right thing, right? It's a cause-and-effect equation: If we want good kids, we should train them up right. And of course, to "train" means to teach and guide someone's actions in the right direction. Most folks I know see this passage as being focused on the end result of the kids, but what if the passage is more of a commentary on the Trainor rather than the Trainee? That is to say, that the admonition might be more directed toward the parent than the child.

Kids model the behavior of their parents. St. Francis of Assisi famously said, "Preach the Gospel at all times. When necessary, use words." Where I come from, we had a saying, "monkey see, monkey do." It's a fair statement that we influence, teach, and instruct more by our behavior than our words. At least it is a much stronger influence. Do as I say, not as I do, is a very poor approach to instruction.

Of course, the message from the pulpit on Sunday when this passage comes up focuses entirely on all the things that none of the parents do, at least obviously. Don't smoke (in public), don't get drunk, don't do drugs, don't have sex outside of marriage, and teach your kids not to do those things either! But have you ever heard a preacher get up and say, "Stop eating yourself to death because your kids are going to do the same thing"? Probably never! Check out what recent health studies are showing:

- An important risk factor for childhood obesity is having parents who are obese. Children with two obese parents are 10 to 20 times more likely to be obese (Reilly) (Whitaker).
- Weight gain in early childhood (3 to 5 years of age) is also significantly greater among children with overweight or obese parents or among those born of overweight or obese mothers (Griffiths).
- Children of heavier parents have been found to exhibit lower levels of physical activity and have a greater preference for high-fat foods and a lower preference for healthier foods (Morgan) (Wardle).
- "Poor-quality diets are now a greater public health threat than malaria, tuberculosis or measles," a new paper by the panel warns. One-in-five deaths are now due to poor diet and that figure is likely to increase. The panel said the growing numbers who are overweight or obese was a particular worry. An estimated 151m children under five – one in four children worldwide – become 'stunted' through poor nutrition. It is not just a matter of height. It leaves them cognitively impaired for life (Food loss & waste, and nutrition).

- Obese children may be less likely to meet a set of five markers for childhood flourishing that include academic and emotional skills, a new analysis of U.S. survey data suggests. Those markers include completing homework, caring about academics, finishing tasks, staying calm when challenged and showing interest in learning, according to the study authors who presented their results on November 3 at the American Academy of Pediatrics annual conference in Orlando, Florida.

Let me boil down the vast amount of research and money spent to arrive at the conclusions of these studies: Train up a child in the way they should go, and when they are older, they won't deviate from your teaching. Yep, if you're fat and live a reckless or uninformed lifestyle, your kids will too. If both Mom and Dad could care less about their health, it's almost guaranteed that the child won't care either. Generational sickness and disease. What a legacy to leave behind!

I guess the question boils down to this: Do you love your kids? If you do, then you will love yourself and teach them to do the same. Allowing them to see you willingly and purposefully kill yourself, slowly over time, is training them to do the same thing, except that the damage to their health starts earlier in their life and is likely to result in a much earlier death.

CHAPTER NINETEEN

The Last Excuse

Now the Spirit expressly says that in later times some will depart from the faith by devoting themselves to deceitful spirits and teachings of demons, through the insincerity of liars whose consciences are seared, who forbid marriage and require abstinence from foods that God created to be received with thanksgiving by those who believe and know the truth. For everything created by God is good, and nothing is to be rejected if it is received with thanksgiving, for it is made holy by the word of God and prayer (1 Tm 4:1-5).

The application of this passage is so abused. I hear it from good-hearted, sincere folks who believe that all foods are OK to eat if you pray over and receive it with thanksgiving. That's not so. Well, perhaps the "food" God created, but certainly not the "food-like" stuff we see today. Let's look at the passage.

First of all, Paul's accusation is toward those with evil intent and that **they** will say that **marriage** and certain food are to be avoided. But Paul says that everything created by God is good. This statement **includes** the covenant of marriage, which God created as He did the food. What forbidden foods are Paul objecting to? The ones "that God created to be received . . ." What were those? Lizards? Vultures? Anything that might have muscle tissue? We've already shown indisputable evidence that God instructed us to eat only those plants and animals that He intended for human consumption. So, is Paul saying that any meat will be OK as long as you pray over it? What about human flesh? Is it OK to eat other people? I mean, when He finished creating man, He said it was good. If being "good" means it's OK to eat, then cannibalism is acceptable, right? That's the logic. How could that be? We get offended at the absurdity of this suggestion, but if you follow the logic that says anything God created is good for food, then that's where you end up. So, that understanding can't be correct, can it? No! The plants and animals that God created for food are acceptable to eat. If you eat some poisonous creature or plant and think you will not die because you prayed over it—you're still going to die.

Furthermore, God didn't create fake food. He's not responsible for the added chemicals that make your body store fat. He didn't put all that sugar in the food he created. In fact, He said too much sugar was a bad thing: It is not good to eat much honey.[2] It's absurd to suggest that God approves of you eating food that you **know** harms your body. Is that what you think this passage is saying? That it's OK to eat whatever you want, knowing that the result will be a significant negative impact on your body, but that's OK with God? Surely not!

Since marriage is also included in the prohibition of some ill-informed people, is Paul saying that **all** marriages are good?

[2] Prv 25:27

Originally, God instituted marriage to be between one man and one woman. Are we to understand that a marriage to a man and child is OK? It is in some cultures, even today. What about in those cultures where men marry men and women marry women? Are all marriages, like all food, now approved? You can't apply the logic unequally in the same verse. I don't believe that God is throwing out His ideals for marriage any more than He is now saying it's OK to eat toxic and poisonous food. To me, that's utter nonsense.

Paul is telling Timothy that there will be fake religious leaders who will begin preaching **lies** that God doesn't approve of marriage and that they shouldn't eat this or that food (which God has already approved) so that the fake religious leaders can restrict their freedom in a way that God never intended.

CHAPTER TWENTY

The Way of Escape

No temptation has overtaken you that is not common to man. God is faithful, and he will not let you be tempted beyond your ability, but with the temptation he will also provide the way of escape, that you may be able to endure it (1 Cor 10:13).

There's a fire in the house! You know this because all the alarm features of your security system are going off, and you can see the smoke and feel the heat from the flames. You have just a few minutes to save your family from being consumed, so what do you do? Do you focus on finding the exit door to safety, or do you give up and allow the fire to consume you?

If you're struggling with the overconsumption or under-consumption of food, your house, God's Temple, is on fire! So now what are you going to do? God has told you that He would provide a way of escape. Are you going to focus on the "way of escape," or will you focus on the problem?

You can tell yourself a thousand times to **stop** doing whatever it is that you shouldn't be doing, and it's not likely going to work because what you've essentially done is refocus your mind **away** from the escape route and back on the problem. There are hundreds of scholarly articles that speak to the effectiveness of focusing your attention on the positive alternative (solution) to your challenge instead of focusing on the problem and its consequences (Forsyth). If it's bad food, start a program and stay focused on following a **good** eating program. If you need to get in shape, focus on getting a health club membership or start a regular walking program, and get some friends to join in. If you need to quit smoking, focus on building other habits that take your mind off smoking. If you're coming up short on money at the end of the month, then focus on adding a revenue stream to your family budget. Wallowing in the embarrassment and disappointment of where you've been isn't going to take you to where you need to be. God, in His great love and mercy, has promised that He'd give you a solution. Spend your time looking for and being focused on the promise of a solution!

I have included an appendix called **Good, Better, Best** at the end of the book. Read it. Pick a solution best suited for you, and by that, I mean something that you will at least try to do. If you make progress on the **Good**, then perhaps you'll move to the **Better**. And once you see the results of that, perhaps you'll move to the **Best**.

Nothing will get you from Point A to Point B overnight. You must move in the right direction and avoid backing up. It took a while for most folks to get their health into questionable, or worse, status. It'll take some time to fix. But, as long as you have time, you have a chance to live the abundant life that you were designed to live.

CHAPTER TWENTY ONE

In Closing

Godly sorrow brings repentance that leads to salvation and leaves no regret, but worldly sorrow brings death (2 Cor 7:10).

Allow me to rephrase: The type of change that God intended is produced through the conviction that one needs to change. Conviction, which is produced by speaking the truth in love, leads to redemption, which revives and rejuvenates a person's spirit with a sense of accomplishment. The type of motivation that the world inflicts on people is through Shame, which humiliates and Condemnation, which rarely produces genuine change.

Shame and Condemnation are poor motivators. Yes, maybe 10% of people would respond positively to that type of motivation, but that means 90% of the people who need to change, even if beaten over the head, will not change. Now, we also must realize that it's often difficult to recognize the internal perception of Conviction versus Shame. Some feel like Condemnation is being heaped on them when it's just the emotional reaction to realizing that they need to make some changes to their lives. Often, especially in the beginning, those pangs of regret and admission are indeed somewhat painful. That doesn't mean that you've been shamed or condemned, but we all need to be careful in how we communicate to one another.

What I like most about this passage is how Paul spells out the human response to proper motivation. Shame and Condemnation don't work. They make a person die a slow death inside. But, when the facts convict someone, and they are lovingly presented and offered a redemptive plan of action, it brings change and peace of mind. Basically, "Here's where you are, here's where you need to be, and here's how to get there." That's a plan.

Now, sometimes the alarm clock goes off and it startles you.

There was a lady we helped whose motivation came from being stuck on a crowded plane. She was taking up her whole seat **and** a portion of the fellow traveler's seat next to her. He complained to the flight attendant in such a way that several rows of people heard him complaining and asking to be seated somewhere else. I can only imagine how embarrassing that must have been. She said it was what motivated her to seek help.

Another person we helped had taken his seat on a roller coaster at an amusement park, but the personnel couldn't get the safety bar to close over the top of him. Out of safety concerns, they wouldn't let the ride begin without the safety bar in its proper position. Unfortunately, there wasn't a discreet way for him to exit, and he had to walk back through the maze of people whom he could hear whispering, "That man was too fat to get on the ride." He said it motivated him to change. Life can be cruel. But that doesn't mean friends should be.

As an example, let's say I have a friend who is overweight by a significant amount. If I say, "Man, I can't believe you've let yourself go like that! You're fat! If you don't care about yourself, you should at least care about your family!" How's that going to be received? But what if I tell that friend, "Hey, you and I both know that your body is telling you that something needs to change or you're going to experience some terrible health consequences. I've got a solution that worked for me. Because you're my friend and I care, I'm willing to lock arms with you to help you find and maintain your very best self." Which do you think is going to work best? Which would you guess would produce change that included a real peace of mind and improved self-esteem?

Shame and Condemnation separate us. Conviction and Redemption draw us closer together and builds community.

> [15]*Look carefully then how you walk, not as unwise but as wise,* [16]*making the best use of the time, because the days are evil.* [17]*Therefore, do not be foolish, but understand what the will of the LORD is* (Eph 5:15-17).

What is the will of God for your life? Maybe it's answered by Jesus Himself.

> *The thief comes only to steal and kill and destroy. I came that they may have life and have it abundantly* (Jn 10:10).

If what you are doing is hurting you, it's of the devil. Jesus came that you could have an abundant life—right here and now.

I can do all things through him who strengthens me (Phil 4:13).

You're able and capable of change.

Mindset is everything for achieving your objectives in life. Paul said, when referring to himself, "I can." He didn't say, "I might," "I will after the holidays," or "I could if this or that were different." No, when it came to how he felt about what God called him to do, he found great confidence in the fact that God was on his side and that anything that needed to be done could be accomplished once he set his mind to do it. What was true for Paul is true for each one of us. Once we make up our minds, the battle is all but won!

It all begins with what you believe to be true: about yourself, about God, and about the power of evil. And what you believe to be true is manifested in how you act. My attitude, my actions, the results I get, and the lifestyle I lead are products of my belief system. What do I believe? How do I act? Same thing.

As a person believes, so they are (Proverbs 23:7, PFV).

You used to be what you once believed; you are presently what you currently believe; you will become what you choose to believe.

Decide today to honor God with your body . . . and you will.

Testimonies of the Saints

*And they have conquered him by the blood of the Lamb
and by the word of their testimony* (Rev 12:11a).

As of the writing of this little book, my wife and I have
helped over 35,000 people worldwide transform their
health to become a more proper expression of their best
selves. I could write many books, if not volumes, recounting
all the various people we have supported through their
transformations: male/female, young/old, overweight/
underweight, athlete/couch potato, etc. But does the Bible
give us any examples? I believe it does, and here are a few.
Undoubtedly, you will think of others who, outside of the
main biblical storyline, demonstrate characteristics, habits,
and patterns of good physical health.

ORIGINAL DESIGN

Let's start with the very first couple: Adam and Eve. If you
want to know what's good for you, then look at what our
Creator designed us all to be entirely dependent on: Air,
Water, Nutrition, Rest, and Social Interaction.

Experts say you can survive approximately three weeks
without food (unless you're Jesus); three days without water;
and three minutes without air. And, while the world record

is around 11 days, most of us can barely think after 24 hours without sleep because our entire body, including our mind, is in shut-down mode. Additionally, most consider total isolation to be a severe form of cruelty and abuse, as severe mental and physical suffering occurs after only a few months.

Then, we see that Adam was instructed to "work and keep" the garden.[3] That is to say, man was created to move rather than sit on his fig leaves. God originally designed Adam and Eve each to live long lives in good health. Genesis 5 tells us that Adam lived for 930 years. Several of the ancient Patriarchs lived very long lives. However, by David's time, our life expectancy was generally around 70 years, and if you took care of yourself, maybe 80.

If you want to live a healthy life, start with clean air, clean water, maximum dense nutrition, proper amounts of sleep, positive social interaction, and physical exercise. It's how God created you to function.

ELISHA'S RUNNING

And the hand of the LORD was on Elijah, and he gathered up his garment and ran before Ahab to the entrance of Jezreel (1 Kgs 18:46).

I suppose that if the hand of the Lord is on you, one can do amazing things. Most of us would **have** to have the hand of the Lord on us to run from Mount Carmel to Jezreel. Depending on which ancient history expert you listen to, this was somewhere between 17-30 miles. In sandals. No Nike running shoes.

---

[3] Gen 2:15

Then, once arriving in Jezreel, our marathon man freaks out in fear of Jezebel and decided to make a run for it . . . all the way to Beersheba. That appears to be approximately 100 miles. In sandals. Then, he leaves his servant (who has been hoofing it across the country with him) behind in Beersheba and heads off by himself on another "day's journey." Historians say that's about 20-25 miles on a good day.

So, Elisha has gone from Mount Carmel to a day's journey outside of Beersheba, or about 150 miles, on foot. In sandals. But he wasn't done yet; however, he was almost physically finished!

Yep, he passed out somewhere in the desert, and an angel had to come to his rescue, bringing food (high carbohydrate and protein cakes), water (hydration), and rest. The Manufacturer knows how to take care of His equipment! However, given the distance and physical exertion that Elisha had expended, he went back to sleep. Once he woke up, the angel made him take in additional food and hydration because he was about to go 40 days and 40 nights (perhaps a figure of speech) to Mount Horeb just on the nutritional support of those two meals! And just so you know, that's approximately another 250 miles! In sandals.

Did God "miraculously" allow Elisha to travel these distances? Maybe. Was Elisha used to traveling by foot? Surely. However, from this narrative, we all should appreciate the importance of nutrition to physical exertion capacity. Whether or not you believe that Elisha was given extraordinary power, his body needed energy and hydration to function properly, which causes me to believe that it wasn't a miracle. The cakes were most likely made from grain flour, which provided protein and carbs for energy.

Water hydrated his body. Rest and recovery were essential. And being properly fueled and recovered, a human body can continue to perform for a good long time without additional energy requirements. It's how we're made. Three meals a day for what most of us are physically required to do? No wonder we as a people are packing on the fat! We don't **need** to eat. We're trained to eat. We want to eat.

WRESTLING WITH JACOB

> [24]*And Jacob was left alone. And a man wrestled with him until the breaking of the day.* [25]*When the man saw that he did not prevail against Jacob, he touched his hip socket, and Jacob's hip was put out of joint as he wrestled with him.* [26]*Then he said, "Let me go, for the day has broken." But Jacob said, "I will not let you go unless you bless me"* (Gen 32:24-26).

You've been traveling with your two wives and the rest of your entourage. You happen across a heavenly being in the evening, so you decide to wrestle with the entity **all night long**. Now, discounting the fact that you're dealing with two wives and family support personnel, and the fact that you can't Uber here or there, along with the obvious confusing decision to want to wrestle with this entity . . . putting all that aside . . . Could you do it?

I've read articles where Olympic athletes couldn't keep up with a 5-year-old for more than half a day, and Jacob wrestles with some heavenly being until the break of day? Could you do that? Yes, I know that the story's point is more focused in another direction, but have we overlooked what Jacob was in physical shape to do? Have we generally ignored the physical preparedness of men and women from these ancient times? Have we relegated being in good physical condition to an earlier time when men and women needed to be in good physical condition? Are we ignoring the need for us to be in good physical condition? How's that working for the average American today? Or for any person in any country who negligently ignores their physical condition? Not so well.

PETER'S SWIM

> [3]*Simon Peter said to them, "I am going fishing." They said to him, "We will go with you." They went out and got into the boat, but that night they caught nothing. -- [7]That disciple whom Jesus loved therefore said to Peter, "It is the Lord!" When Simon Peter heard that it was the Lord, he put on his outer garment, for he was stripped for work, and threw himself into the sea. [8]The other disciples came in the boat, dragging the net full of fish, for they were not far from the land, but about a hundred yards off* (Jn 21:3, 7-8).

You've been up all night fishing. Not with some Zebco spinning outfit but with nets—big nets—flung into the water and then hauled back up every so often. That's **work**. Hard work! And now some guy on the shore tells you how to fish! You're about ready to row over there and give him a piece of your mind until your fishing buddy tells you it's Jesus. You do the only reasonable thing: you put on your robe and jump in and swim to shore! What?!?

The text says they are a hundred yards offshore. That's about three city blocks or down and back in an Olympic-sized pool. When's the last time you swam a hundred yards? When's the last time you did it in your bathrobe? The robe's weight and the restriction must have added a ton of resistance to the swim, but Peter was fired up. Fired up or not, that took a tremendous amount of effort, and remember it was after a night on the boat trying to catch fish with nets. Say what you will about Peter's personality quirks; he was apparently in fantastic physical shape.

ESTHER'S MAKEOVER

So when the king's order and his edict were proclaimed, and when many young women were gathered in Susa the citadel in custody of Hegai, Esther also was taken into the king's palace and put in custody of Hegai, who had charge of the women. And the young woman pleased him and won his favor. And he quickly provided her with her cosmetics and her portion of food, and with seven chosen young women from the king's palace, and advanced her and her young women to the best place in the harem (Est 2:8-9).

We've read a lot about the men, but what about the experiences of the women? My wife reminded me of Esther and her physical transformation that took a year to complete.

In this book of the Bible, we learn that all the women who were rounded up to be considered worthy of belonging in the king's harem weren't just washed and fluffed. The king put them through a year-long process of being physically transformed. The text mentions two areas of concern: the consumption of food and the treatment of the skin.

I find it interesting that the ancient civilizations knew how to improve one's appearance by natural means. The text says this: Now when the turn came for each young woman to go in to King Ahasuerus, after being twelve months under the regulations for the women, since this was the regular period of their beautifying, six months with oil of myrrh and six months with spices and ointments for women.[4]

A six-month treatment with oil of myrrh and another six-month treatment with spices and ointments **for women** (I suppose they were the first to have developed their own "men's line"). Note also that, as part of this year-long "beautifying," the women were provided with **their portion** of food. This wasn't some spa with an all-you-can-eat buffet at the king's palace! No, the ancients knew that to look your best, you had to take care of your skin **and** eat the appropriate amount of food. The royals passed this idea of beauty treatment down to present-day people, and today the global beauty industry is valued at around $500 **billion**, which includes products for men and women (Cvetkovska). The health and wellness industry was worth $4.5 **trillion** in 2018 (McGroarty). That's trillion with a T. The truth is—we know how to take care of our bodies. We have for a long, long time.

So, the questions are: Ladies, do you care for your skin occasionally, or do you make it a regular daily practice? Do you use skincare and beauty products that are natural and healthy or those that contain harsh chemicals that damage your body? Are you aware of what a "portion" of food is for you, and do you exercise restraint to abide by it most of the time? When's the last time you spent time "beautifying" yourself?

Just because we're focused on Esther doesn't mean I'm excluding the men here. Men don't have to look like a Shar-Pei dog or the rugged Marlboro man anymore. The worn-out leather look is out of style. You don't have to

---

[4] Est 2:12

smell like a petunia to take care of your skin and put forth a healthy appearance. Maybe your "Esther" would appreciate the effort you put forth into taking care of your skin **and** understanding that you should limit your food consumption to **your** portion and not that of three men!

I've heard it said that the majority of new enrollees at health clubs are those who have broken up with their boy/girlfriend or have recently divorced. It's common to get complacent and take things and people for granted. Maybe, just maybe, if spouses stayed in reasonably good health and physical appearance, there wouldn't be a 50% divorce rate in America. I don't know. Just throwing it out there.

PAUL

So many books have been written about the life and times of the Apostle Paul that it's difficult to include him without feeling a bit intimidated, but I'm not going to tackle the theology and inspiration of this great man. I'm going to briefly mention his physicality.

Paul went on three missionary journeys between AD 46-57 and was taken to Rome in AD 60. The distance has been calculated, and although I'm sure there is a range of distances according to the person doing the measuring, I'm sure you'll agree that the journeys were a **long way**!

The first missionary journey was measured at 1,581 miles.

The second journey was 3,050 miles.

The third journey was 3,307 miles.

His journey to Rome was 2,344 miles.

That's over 10,000 miles by foot, animal, and boat. Forget 10,000 steps on a Fitbit; this was 10,000 **miles**! You don't travel 10,000 miles in those days and in that manner without being in a state of good health. But that shouldn't surprise you about Paul. He often mentions physical activity.

> [24]*Do you not know that in a race all the runners run, but only one receives the prize? So run that you may obtain it.* [25]*Every athlete exercises self-control in all things. They do it to receive a perishable wreath, but we an imperishable.* [26]*So I do not run aimlessly; I do not box as one beating the air.* [27]*But I discipline my body and keep it under control, lest after preaching to others I myself should be disqualified* (1 Cor 9:24-27).

In just this one small part of his letter to the Corinthians he mentions competitive running, athletes' disciplined training, boxing, and his personal physical disciplines. Yes, Paul was a Type-A personality, but the inspiration of the letter should inform you that being in good shape physically is preferable to the alternative!

In another letter to Timothy, Paul says this: *for while bodily training is of some value, godliness is of value in every way, as it holds promise for the present life and also for the life to come* (1 Tm 4:8).

If you read this and think, "See? Physical activity is of little value," then you're missing the point. No, nothing we do is of greater value than living a life of godliness in every aspect of one's life, but honoring God with your body is a command and is part of that life dedicated to following the procedures outlined in The Owner's Manual! Yes, bodily training is of significant value both physically and spiritually, and each of us should incorporate some activity based on our abilities.

PEOPLE I'VE KNOWN

We could go on and on talking about the various people in the Bible who demonstrated tremendous physical strengths, but what about people today? Glad you asked.

Here are just a few examples of the over 35,000 people that my wife and I have helped transform.[5]

Africa - Over 600 lbs. and in hospice. You don't go to hospice to recover. She was the first person in my experience whose primary motivation to transform was **not to die**! A neighbor who went to visit with her almost every day finally talked her into trying to recover. She lost her husband, her folks were divvying up her assets, and she was just about to turn out the lights when she decided to change. Two years later, she's in her skinny jeans and fully recovered. She lost over 450 pounds. She doesn't plan on looking for it either!

Lancelot - Outdoorsman. Loved to hunt and fish. He loved to take his kids with him into the great outdoors and teach them about the wonders of nature, but he had gotten so overweight that he couldn't get out much. His identity as an outdoorsman was dying, and he wanted to change. 90 pounds later, he was running to his deer stand. Pictures of him taking his kids hunting and fishing were back on Facebook.

Judy - Judy was sick and in bed. She didn't have the energy to get out of bed and was **underweight** and not eating. Judy was really sick. She kind of freaked out on us when we got

---

[5] Names have been changes to protect their privacy.

her started with nutrition. She didn't want to be on a "diet" because she was already severely underweight. But she trusted us and got started. Judy was working in her flower garden within days. Judy got back to her healthy weight, and her energy went through the roof. Nutrition isn't about losing weight. It's about fueling yourself with what God intended you to use as fuel to operate at maximum efficiency.

Rosemary - Rosemary was overweight as a kid. She was overweight as an adult. She said the hateful comments she experienced as she went from adolescent to teenager to young adult emotionally scarred her. She tried diet after diet to no avail and had decided that she would be obese for the rest of her life. She was cursed, big-boned, genetically inferior—her list went on and on. Rosemary is no longer obese. Nutrition and intermittent fasting changed her life. She's not an inferior product, but a child of the Most-High God who needed direction.

I could go on for days talking about the men and women, the elderly and the teenagers, the folks of all races and many heritages, the pro athletes, the college athletes, the Olympic athletes, the coach potatoes. I could talk about those that have extra challenges with their health who, unfortunately, must try harder to get the same results.

It doesn't matter if you're underweight, overweight, short, tall, from New York, Arkansas, or Taiwan; there is likely no challenge that you're facing that somebody hasn't already faced and won. All it took for those other people to succeed was an honest accounting of where they stood, a determination to change, and a reliable method which they followed. Just don't wait too long.

The Bible is an amazing story of God's redemption of

humankind. But, at some point, the opportunity to change ends. The words to an old hymn written by George F. Root come to mind, and I'll leave it with you as I close.

"Why do you wait, dear brother?
The harvest is passing away;
Your Savior is longing to bless you;
There's danger and death in delay."

Why not, why not, why not come to Him now?

Good, Better, Best

First, I think it's important to communicate that fad diets are not a long-term solution to your health. Nobody stays on a "diet" for very long. Almost all of them are based on carbohydrate restriction so severe that most people can't do it for very long. When people restrict carbs, their metabolism, the fat burning process of the body, has slowed so dramatically that when they stop their "diet" and eat a peanut butter and jelly sandwich, they gain back five pounds!

Other plans have you chopping and cutting and measuring and weighing. If your plan isn't something that you can continue for the rest of your life, don't do it.

Another unfortunate recommendation is what some of us call the "Push Away" diet—often recommended by medical professionals with little to no training in nutrition, especially as a remedial intervention into health issues. Essentially, the admonition is to "push away" from the table and get some exercise. The difficulty is that people who are basically malnourished (one can be skinny or obese and still be malnourished) who have a very poor diet are told to eat less of the food they presently eat that contains very little actual nutrition and are encouraged to put their bodies through rigorous exercise. It is rarely successful because the extra exertion recommended requires nutrients to fuel it, and you don't have it to spare. You tire easily, recover slowly, you'll be so sore you can't walk up the stairs or comb your hair, and you will quit quickly. If someone recommends this diet to you, nod politely and leave.

For those of you, like me, who have an elementary understanding of nutrition and how it works, let me share the illustration that my nutritional guru and good friend, Stephen Ashcraft, shared with me.

Your body is like a computer. Everybody is somewhat familiar with a computer, right? Three things make a computer function properly: Energy, Operating System, and Programs. Simply put, electricity is the energy. Windows 10 is my operating system, and Microsoft Word is the program I'm using to type this page. Are you with me so far? Now, here's the correlation.

The energy needed by your body (computer) is carbohydrates, protein, and fat. They power the body. Vitamins, minerals, trace minerals, etc., make up the operating system. They allow the body to operate its various functions, just as Windows allows my laptop to operate Microsoft Word. The programs are my brain, heart, lungs, digestion, muscular frame, bones, etc. For my programs to function properly, I must have the power and the operating system in proper working order. And I must be careful not to allow viruses, malware, and clutter to enter the operating system, causing everything to slow down and function poorly. Make sense?

One thing that a laptop or iPad will do is store excess energy in a battery in case you need it later. The body does the same thing. The only difference is that the laptop battery only has so much storage capacity and will quit storing or using excess energy when the battery is full. The body has nearly an unlimited ability to store excess energy as fat cells. It'll keep making new cells to store energy as long as there is excess coming in. When the power is cut off, the body uses the excess stored energy. That's how it works in a nutshell.

But like who has time to be a nutritionist? The science of nutrition can be overwhelming, confusing, and, as is often the case, professionals differ in their opinions. Some plans and recommendations can be **expensive,** and while some work for a short period, they aren't lifestyle choices! So, here are three ideas to get you headed in the right direction. Remember, before starting any plan, you should check with your physician to make sure you won't die. That's the proverbial disclaimer.

GOOD

A "good" thing to do as a beginner is to **stop** eating foods that are bad for you. A general rule of thumb is to stop eating "white" foods such as white bread, refined white sugar, white pasta, and white potatoes.

These items are loaded with "energy" that you don't need. They make batteries the size of your living room, but you don't need that much energy to run your computer. Stop plugging into these high energy sources.

Stop the habit of having dessert after all your meals.

Stop drinking so much. Alcohol converts to sugar. Sugar is energy. We've covered that.

Stop buying highly processed snack foods. Nibbling is a polite expression for grazing. If you look at the bag and you can't understand what's in it, don't eat it.

Stop eating so much. I know, your momma told you to clean your plate because of all those starving kids in some far-off land, but you shouldn't eat until you're gorged. Try and practice some portion control and slow down.

If you **stop** some of the bad habits you've developed over time, you'll see real improvement in how you feel and look.

Let me throw in something here on sugar since they load most of the awful things we eat with sugar. My guess is that many of you won't know this.

Many health professionals believe that sugar is as addictive, or nearly as addictive, as cocaine (Schaefer). Yes, you read that right. Sugar causes changes in the brain that are very similar to that of other highly addictive substances. That's great for the sugar industry but horrible for you. When starting a reduced-calorie plan, people will often experience a sugar "withdrawal." Fortunately, it's not nearly as intense or long-lasting, but it's noticeable.

Nobody knows how much sugar they eat. Do you keep up with counting every gram of sugar in everything you eat? Not likely. If you spent just a couple of days keeping up with it, you'd find out that the amount of sugar you eat is astounding. It's in everything!

Two hundred years ago, the average American ate only two pounds of sugar a year. In 1970, we ate 123 pounds of sugar per year. Today, the average American consumes almost 152 pounds of sugar in one year. This is equal to three pounds (or six cups) of sugar consumed in one week! Nutritionists suggest that Americans should get only 10% of their calories from sugar. This equals 13.3 teaspoons of sugar per day (based on 2,000 calories per day). The current average is 42.5 teaspoons of sugar per day (How much sugar do you eat? You may be suprised!).

Another somewhat deceptive practice is the lack of "recommended daily allowance" (RDA) listed on nutritional labels for sugar. Everything else on the label will indicate what that particular food item has in terms of nutrient value and what percentage it takes up of the RDA for that nutrient . . . except sugar. Look on the labels. Everything else has a value attached to it except sugar. Why? Because the FDA couldn't establish what was and what was not a "safe" level of consumption when they established labeling requirements in the 1990s. It's fair to say that the sugar industry had a voice in that debate. However, more and more professionals expressed concerns for more transparency, given the additional research by professionals on sugar consumption. After much effort and political posturing, the FDA is adopting new requirements, which will provide more transparency to the consumer (Mayne).

Another **good** thing to do is monitor how much you're spending on food. Most folks don't really know. We know how much we spent at the grocery store, but do you know what you spent for breakfast, lunch, and snacks? Most people spend somewhere between $12-20 per day per person.

Disclaimer: It's not what you do 10% of the time that's causing you to gain weight, feel sluggish, and generally have your health "cart" in the ditch. It's what you do 90% of the time. When Ms. Smith brings out her soon-to-be world-famous banana pudding or Aunt Jean brings her coconut cake to the family reunion, go ahead and have some. Life is meant to be lived. But life is meant to be lived well, so don't eat the whole thing. Enjoy yourself, but have some self-discipline and restraint. It'll pay off big time.

To sum up good: Stop eating things that are not good for you. You'll likely save some money, lose some weight, and feel much better.

BETTER

Once you've established **good** habits, take it up a notch. None of us start out being health-junkies, but we begin by incorporating healthy habits into our lifestyle a little at a time. It's easier to do, and we build lasting lifestyle habits. So, what are some **better** ideas?

As discussed above, eliminating certain food items is extremely beneficial, but a **better** plan would be to **add in** certain food items and nutrients that are beneficial. You've heard the expression, "out with the old and in with the new?" That's doing **better**.

Fresh fruits and vegetables should be a daily addition to your consumption habits. The fresher, the better. Organic is good for some things if it's not overly pricey. If you're fortunate to have a local farmer's market where locally grown items are available, go there! These fresh fruits and veggies are essential to providing the daily nutrients you need in order for your "programs" to run more efficiently.

Try to choose lean meats like chicken and fish and back off on some of the red meat. Try baked, broiled, or grilled instead of deep-fried! Be creative and have fun coming up with healthy food ideas. If eating healthy meant everything had to taste like kale, none of us would do it. Fortunately, there are some great ideas out there. Have you tried the cauliflower rice? Oh, man!

Drink more water and for heaven's sake, avoid carbonated beverages like soda.

Get more sleep. Stress is a killer, and getting plenty of rest will help with your stress levels.

Once you've checked with your doctor to make sure you won't die, add some basic exercise, like walking, to your daily regimen. You don't have to walk a long way. However, you should be consistent. Whether it's two or three times per week or every day, do it. If you're capable, then get your butt to the gym and get your cardio and resistance training in. An investment in your health is an investment in the most important thing in your life after your relationship with Jesus.

Another recommendation comes from being involved in the health and wellness field for the past 15 years. Establish an accountability partner. Whether you're doing this together or you just want your partner to hold you accountable, having at least one supportive person around you is very helpful.

Establish a goal. Everybody needs to have a plan of action. Write down what you'd like to accomplish, put a date on it by which you want to reach your goal, and then share it with your accountability partner. And quit worrying about failure. The first time you brushed your teeth, it was a disaster, but I bet you've got it down pretty well by now.

BEST

The very best exercise is the one you'll do consistently; however, it's commonly accepted that H.I.I.T. (High Intensity Interval Training) will give you the most bang for your buck as it relates to burning fat and overall conditioning. You better make sure you've checked with somebody to make sure you will not die. It's a heart-pounding experience.

The very best food choices are less of what you've been conditioned to believe is "food" and more of what is a known quantity of the exact vitamins, minerals, trace minerals, etc., with the optimum amount of protein, carbs, and fat. It's often referred to as "dense nutrition." You're packing in all the nutrients that the Good Lord designed you to have and use in an ideal caloric vehicle.

You could go out to a grocery store, farmer's market, or local seller and hand-select the best you could find, and you'd still not have a clue what kind of overall nutrition you'd be receiving. You could come close to getting what you need daily, but it'd be lucky if you did, and it'd be very costly. I recommend involving yourself in a program that does all the formulation for you in a cost-effective manner without sacrificing anything on quality. But do your research because not all products and not all companies are the same. Yes, you can enjoy "regular" food, but your focus should be on nutrition at this point in your wellness journey. You already have adjusted in the **better** category for eating the "right" foods, so work on nutrition. It makes all the difference in how you feel, and once you feel like a million bucks, you won't make the decision to go back to the way you used to feel.

Another tremendously beneficial activity is nutritionally supported intermittent fasting. We were originally defined as "hunter-gatherers." We hunted what was available and harvested fruits and vegetables in season. Since there wasn't much in terms of our ability to preserve food, we ate it when we had it and went looking for it when we didn't. There were days that early man didn't eat. Rather than being harmful, modern medicine has proven that a nutritionally supported and time-limited fast can have tremendous benefits to your system, especially in the support of your body's natural elimination of toxins, the release of excess energy (fat), and several other benefits. Persons with diabetic issues can also fast, but they also have to pay closer attention to their blood sugar levels. It's one of the healthiest things that you can do physically and mentally. You learn to control your hunger, and controlling what you do is ultimately where we all wish to get to.

The Bible treats fasting as a spiritual cleansing process, but what we've learned is that health benefits from physical cleansing are also substantial.

The only other **best** recommendation I would add to the mix is to continue improving your focus on health and wellness. I'm fortunate to have a good friend who I call my "nutritional guru." He knows more about this sort of thing than anybody I know. The only challenge is trying to get him to give me just a "nickel's worth" when he's got a $100 worth of knowledge. I mean, there's only so much I can absorb! With all the "latest and greatest" fad diets coming out, you must be able to trust someone to steer you in the right direction. This could be an author, a holistic medical professional, a nutritionist, or perhaps even the organization where you prefer to get your daily nutritional supplies. The point is, if you're not an expert, you need to educate yourself on what you're putting in your body.

It reminds me of an ancient Chinese proverb: I hear and I forget; I see and I remember; I do and I understand. Benjamin Franklin is attributed with later saying, "Tell me and I forget, teach me and I may remember, involve me and I learn." It's one thing to know, another thing to remember, and quite another thing to learn. Now that you know what the Bible says about taking care of yourself, you need to do it. Decide that you want to honor God with your body, and you'll do exactly that.

Best of success.

For more information on how to design a personalized plan of action please contact the author at:

R. Price Futrell, Independent Associate,
Isagenix International

pricefutrell@gmail.com
www.watchthevideo.info

References

"Chemical Use in Animal Production: Issues and Alternatives." University of California, Agricultural Issues Center, 1989. <https://aic.ucdavis.edu/publications/oldanrpubs/chemicalsanimals.pdf>.

Cho, Sungsoo et al. "The effect of breakfast type on total daily energy intake and body mass index: results from the Third National Health and Nutrition Examination Survey (NHANES III)." *Journal of the American College of Nutrition* 22,4 (2003): 296-302.

Cvetkovska, Ljubica. "45 Beauty Industry Statistics That Will Impress You." 8 January 2019. *loudcloudhealth.com.*

Davis, Donald R et al. "Changes in USDA food composition data for 43 garden crops, 1950 to 1999." *Journal of the American College of Nutrition* 23,6 (2004): 669-82. Website.

Davis, Donald R. "Declining Fruit and Vegetable Nutrient Composition: What Is the Evidence?" *HortScience horts* 44,1 (2009): 15-19. Web. <https://doi.org/10.21273/HORTSCI.44.1.15>.

Dodor, Bernice. "The Impact of Religiosity on Health Behaviors and Obesity among African Americans." *Journal of Human Behavior in the Social Environment* 22,4 (2012): 451-462.

Forsyth, Jennifer K., et al. "Augmenting NMDA receptor signaling boosts experience-dependent neuroplasticity in the adult human brain." *Proceedings of the National Academy of Sciences* 112, 50 (2015): 15331-15336.

Gillum, R. Frank. "Frequency of Attendance at Religious Services, Overweight, and Obesity in American Women and Men: The Third National Health and Nutrition Examination Survey." *Annals of Epidemiology* 16.9 (2006): 655-660. <http://www.sciencedirect.com/science/article/pii/S1047279705003790>.

Griffiths, L J et al. "Risk factors for rapid weight gain in preschool children: findings from a UK-wide prospective study." *International journal of obesity (2005)* 34,4 (2010): 624-32.

"How much sugar do you eat? You may be suprised!" August 2014. *New Hampshire Department of Health and Human Services.*

Link, Rachael. "8 Health Benefits of Fasting, Backed by Science." 30 July 2018. *healthline.*

Mayne, Susan T. "Statement on new guidance for the declaration of added sugars on food labels for single-ingredient sugars and syrups and certain cranberry products." 18 June 2019. *U.S. Food & Drug Administration.*

McGroarty, Beth. "WELLNESS INDUSTRY STATISTICS & FACTS." n.d. *globalwellnessinstitute.org.*

Morgan, Philip J et al. "Correlates of objectively measured physical activity in obese children." *Obesity (Silver Spring, Md.)* 16,12 (2008): 2634-41.

Reilly, John J, et al. "Early life risk factors for obesity in childhood: cohort study." *BMJ* 330,7504 (2005): 1357. Document.

Wardle, J et al. "Food and activity preferences in children of lean and obese parents." *International journal of obesity and related metabolic disorders : journal of the International Association for the Study of Obesity* 25,7 (2001): 971-7.

Whitaker, Katriina L et al. "Comparing maternal and paternal intergenerational transmission of obesity risk in a large population-based sample." *The American journal of clinical nutrition* 91,6 (2010): 1560-7.

Endnotes

[i] Price Futrell Version
[ii] Scripture quotations are taken from the English Standard Version (ESV).

Thank You

Thank You For Reading My Book!

I really appreciate all of your feedback, and I love hearing what you have to say.

I need your input to make the next version of this book and my future books even better.

Please leave me a helpful review on Amazon letting me know what you thought of the book.

Thank you so much!
R. Price Futrell

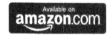

Made in United States
North Haven, CT
13 April 2023

35413792R00075